We Will Meet Again in Heaven

We Will Meet Again in Heaven

CHRISTEL AND ISABELL ZACHERT

Translated by Stephen Trobisch

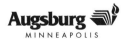

Augsburg

MINNEAPOLIS

WE WILL MEET AGAIN IN HEAVEN

English translation copyright © 1995 Augsburg Fortress

Translated from *Wir treffen uns wieder in meinem Paradies*, © 1993
by Gustav Lübbe Verlag GmbH, Bergisch Gladbach.

Cover design by Brad D. Norr/Minneapolis

Library of Congress Cataloging-in-Publication Data

Zachart, Christel.
   [Wir treffen uns wieder in meinem paradies. English]
   We will meet again in heaven : one family's remarkable struggle
with death and life / Christel and Isabell Zachert : translated by
Stephen Trobisch.
     p.   cm.
   Translation of: Wir treffen uns wieder in meinem paradies.
   ISBN 0–8066–2752–2
   1. Zachert, Isabell, 1966–1982—health. 2. Cancer in children—
Patients—Germany—Biography. 3. Cancer in children—Patients—
Family relationships. 4. Cancer—Religious aspects—Christianity. I.
Zachert, Isabell, 1966–1982. II. Title.
   RC281.C4Z33913 1995
   362.1'9892994'00092—dc20   95-11807
                                         [B]CIP

The paper used in this publication meets the minimum requirements
of American National Standard for Information Services—Permanence
of Paper for Printed Library Materials, ANSI Z329.48-1984.   ∞

Manufactured in the U.S.A.   AF 9-2752
99 98 97 96 95 1 2 3 4 5 6 7 8 9 10

I dedicate this book to my husband and our two sons
Christian and Matthias. I wish to thank Doctor
Töbellius for his friendship and Frau Von Löbbecke
for her motherly care.

CHRISTEL ZACHERT

I wish to thank my wife Kim for her assistance
with the translation. She helped me more than I can say.

STEPHEN TROBISCH

Ten Years Later

MY DEAR DAUGHTER,

I arrived in the Ardennes at the vacation home of a dear friend. Now I look forward to being with you in spirit and to sharing thoughts. Here I have the peace and quiet to let myself go in the memories of your last months.

Ten years ago you went ahead of us—into heaven. And you were right: we have not lost you. Your confidence and strength have supported and protected us so much! In the hours of your unconsciousness preceding your death, I read for the first time your diary of the last weeks of your life. I read it aloud to all for whom you had written it. Since then it has been my deep desire to share this legacy with others. I am sure this is your wish too.

I hope to find the strengthening well of memory rather than the inconsolable valley of tears. The circumstances are favorable for me. I feel safe with a caring friend. You did not know her, but I have told her about you. She supported my writing plans and invited me to her vacation home in the Ardennes. She provides for my physical well-being and sees to it that I do not get lost with my thoughts in the valley of tears.

I will try to walk through the most intense year of my life by following my heart. It was your last year—the fifteenth and sixteenth year of your life. It was a year of highlights as well as unspeakable pain, a year full of enticing hope and deepest despair. In spite of all hardship it was a year of wonderment for all of us. Within one year we saw you change from a young, happy, normal girl into a mature woman. All the doctors, nurses, and everyone who took part in your—in our—destiny, were attracted by your strength. It was by the mercy of God that you died like a princess, consciously saying goodbye to all your loved ones and even arranging the farewell celebration yourself.

Let us begin then! I want to attempt it. If the Lord asks me some day how I used the gift of life, I don't want to stand in front of God with an excuse. Part of the gift of life for me is sharing everything you have given to us through your life and death.

Your father and I had come back from Rome. We had taken our first trip without our children. You and your brothers, Christian and Matthias, were proud to be left alone for a whole week. We felt that we had arrived at a new phase in our marriage. Enriched with beautiful impressions and fulfilled with great joy, we returned home.

It was a Saturday evening. We wanted to be back in time for Matthias' fourteenth birthday. Christian and Matthias greeted us happily, but they told us that you had already gone to bed and that you were asleep. That surprised us, but we respected it.

After a while you woke up. You came out of your room looking pale and exhausted like someone who is very ill. We tried to comfort you. On Sunday morning Dad took you to our family doctor. He said you had a lingering influenza infection and prescribed penicillin. He recommended an X-ray of your lungs after the fever subsided.

On Sunday we were busy telling about our trip to Rome and asking about your health. We thought that something was causing your severe "influenza." You had gone to a party, but that couldn't have been the cause. Two days earlier you were at the sports club, where you swam two thousand meters, went to the sauna, and returned home on your bicycle. Maybe it was the bicycle, the old one-speed bicycle that is so hard to ride—maybe that was to blame. (Matthias still treasures that old bicycle, which he uses to get to the university.) On Sunday you said something that kept troubling us: "If I'm sick then I'm really sick, and I have been for a long time."

On Monday and Tuesday your fever subsided, but you grew weaker and weaker. A lump began to show on your ribs, and because it wasn't black and blue, we couldn't explain it. (On a field trip four weeks earlier you had been bumped on that spot.) Wednesday you had increasing difficulties speaking. You sat up in bed gasping for air. I called Dad, who came from work, and we took you to the hospital. We suspected that you had pneumonia.

Right after the X-ray exam of your lungs we were told that your life was in acute danger. You had to be treated immediately in the hospital. The senior physician was

9

called. Your lungs had to be tapped immediately or you would suffocate. We did not leave you for a moment. We saw that the fluid taken from your lungs was red.

When Dr. Petri inserted the second cannula, he sent the first one back to the lab for further analysis. Then he called the director of the hospital, Dr. Töbellius, and said: "There is a young woman here who I believe will be of interest to you." They treated you with great concentration and care, but they gave us no explanation. Dad and I tried to stay calm. You were quite brave. They had to draw at least two or three cannulas of fluid from your lungs to prevent a circulatory collapse. In the meantime a bed was prepared for you in a hospital room with another young girl.

After we made sure that you were taken care of, we looked for the doctors. We found Dr. Petri in the lab and asked him directly for his opinion. He told us frankly that you had a malignant tumor and that it was in its final stage. It was still too early to determine the type of tumor.

We were shocked but tried to maintain our composure. An experience, twenty-two years before, came instantly to my mind: doctors informed my mother and us four children—I was nineteen years old at the time—that our mother had a tumor in her lungs and that not even a miracle of God's grace would save her. She died two weeks later.

Now I understood the seriousness of your situation, as well as our own. We did not want our fears to enter your heart. You needed all your strength to deal with your pain and burden. We were not yet able to tell you what we already knew.

We had planned this day to be very happy. Grandma—Dad's mother—returned on this day from her trip to Japan. We had planned to pick her up from the airport and celebrate her return. Without leaving the hospital, we rearranged everything. In the evening, when you were exhausted and tired, we finally did see Grandma. As I recall, we did not yet mention the word tumor to her, but we told her you had a very serious illness.

After visiting with Grandma, we stopped by the hospital. A young man was on night duty. He offered to let us see you, but we didn't have the courage. For a few minutes we stood in front of your door. The young man comforted us and told us you were asleep. When we came back home, we gave a brief account to the boys. Matthias and Christian were stunned. They couldn't understand what had happened to you and didn't know what lay ahead of them. I sensed that this was the last day of their childhood and youth!

As we tried to figure out what we should say to you and to other people, Dad and I cried. Finally we fell asleep.

The next day was another busy one. All kinds of medical technologies were used for further examinations. We were asked to collect all your medical records, X-rays, and examination reports, of which there were quite a few. Your last exam had been only four weeks earlier and included an X-ray of your ribs and a complete blood profile. You were examined because of your complaints after the boat trip on the Dutch canals with your school class. When you returned, you complained of a sharp pain in your ribs on your right side, so we sent you to our family doctor. Fortunately your ribs were not fractured, and everything seemed to be all right.

11

Then there were all the reports about your ankle surgery. That previous summer you had an injury that was so painful that the university clinic as well as Dr. Dederich recommended surgery. For you this operation was serious because it limited your capacity for sports and physical movement. The worst part for you was not being allowed to play tennis anymore; you were such an enthusiastic tennis player! I still keep your trophies in a display case. You were also forbidden to jog, which was hard for you to accept. When your cast was removed, you gradually started to swim and bike again. But that still wasn't enough to guarantee your future happiness. How much we still needed to learn to accept small gains.

We even obtained the records of 1968 from the children's clinic. You had survived a nearly fatal fall at the age of two. We cared for you for three months until you recovered from a concussion. At that time we felt God had given us our daughter back again.

So we did collect all your medical reports, but I don't think they helped the doctors much.

By the afternoon the doctors had learned that the cancer had already spread throughout your body, but we didn't know that yet. In the evening Dr. Töbellius visited you with the chief surgeon to examine your ribs. I observed both doctors. They did not talk but communicated only by eye contact. At the end of the exam the surgeon touched your back almost lovingly and he silently uttered the word "full." At that moment I knew his diagnosis. The doctors decided to perform a biopsy to obtain a tissue sample for determining the type of tumor. First your lungs had to be drained by inserting a catheter. That took several days.

On Friday, for the first time, we had a long conversation with Dr. Töbellius. He was very understanding. From a medical point of view the diagnosis was, as I suspected, hopelessly grim. You had a sarcoma, a tumor in the connective tissue, and a very aggressive one. Dr. Töbellius, however, tried to leave us some reason to hope.

I asked him: "How long will Isabell live?" He did not answer. I kept on pushing: "If our daughter continues to decline at this rate, she won't live for five days." He just looked at me with his big brown eyes. I knew that he was thinking in terms of only a few days. This was the standard prognosis—unless there was a miracle. Dr. Töbellius did, however, implant faith in us, faith in such a miracle. And what was much more important: he made it clear to us that we needed to transmit this faith to you. From that day on we felt a deep trust in this man.

The biopsy was supposed to take place Monday. We did not leave you for a single minute. You had many visitors. Everyone wanted to see you one more time. Fortunately this kept you so busy that you did not have time to ask us any questions.

On Saturday afternoon my youngest brother, Siegfried, came from Mannheim to visit you in the hospital. He brought his wife, Ulli, and their little daughter, Sascha, who was only four weeks old. He had to try hard to hold back his tears. As always, he brought his camera. In that way he could hide behind the camera so you couldn't read his eyes. You had a lot of fun with little Sascha. Holding a tiny baby in your arms seemed wonderful for you, a symbol of life. Siegfried and Ulli hoped some of the strength of this young life could be transferred to you.

You began to write letters. By Friday you already finished a letter to your godmother Ines. For a long time you had been close to her. She had been suffering from cancer for half a year.

Dear Ines,

I am back in the hospital again—but let me tell you one thing at a time.

You may know that my parents went to Rome for a week. They used Rolli's empty apartment, because he had just left for the United States.

They left with friends by car on the 29th, and they handed over all the responsibility to us children. There were five of us:

1. The three of us (Christian, Matthias, and I).

2. Marie, the maid who is staying with us for one year. She is a French-speaking Belgian. We get along fine. She's twenty.

3. Caroline Hopchet, a friend from Belgium. I visited her family during my fall break.

I had to take charge, because Christian and Matthias didn't and because it is not fair to make a guest responsible. Marie helped me a lot though.

Each day during that week it was harder for me to breathe. I didn't go to the doctor, because I thought that it was just bronchitis—and besides I had to take care of the apartment and the boys. Friday Caroline and Marie left. During the week, Caroline went with me to school.

*Saturday I cleaned the apartment, and in the evening
our parents returned from Rome. They were full of stories
about their trip.*

*I guess I gave them a big scare. I must have been white
as a sheet. I staggered around and gasped for air.*

*Dad immediately took me to our family doctor on
Sunday morning. She said that I had pneumonia in its
early stage. The fever subsided, and everything got better,
except I had trouble breathing and my right shoulder hurt
no matter how I sat or lay. Our family doctor had arranged
an X-ray appointment at the hospital for Wednesday afternoon. As soon as I was X-rayed, they told us that my life
was in danger because my entire right lung was filled with
fluid, which put pressure on my heart and left lung. They
kept me at the hospital to drain my lung. Thursday they
performed more tests to find out the cause. They also
drained some fluid from my spinal cord by using a syringe,
and on Friday they inserted a permanent catheter between
the lung and the pleura.*

*I never thought that anything so awful would happen
to me.*

*Everyone here in the hospital is tremendously nice. I
have been to the hospital quite often, but no other hospital
has been so pleasant.*

*Grandma came back from Japan on Wednesday and
brought beautiful things for every one of us. For Bolko,
my uncle, she brought a Walkman—a small cassette
player with headphones—and yesterday he gave it to me
as a present. That's really nice! Mom and Dad come to
see me often, and so do Christian and Matthias. So far I
have about seven visitors per day, and one day I even had
fifteen. Everyone is so kind to me.*

I get a lot of compliments on the watch you gave me.
Every day I'm happy to have it.
Greetings and kisses to all your loved ones. All the best
to you, my dear Ines.

Your "Hospital Belli"

P.S. I can't write very well because I am having a lot of pain.

The biopsy was performed on Monday. Fortunately your system tolerated the anesthesia well. After the operation you were given a single room, and the nurses put up a second bed for us. That way Dad or I could stay with you overnight. Now Dad and I had to collect our thoughts. It was a time of intense conversations, deep thoughts, and darkest nightmares. Could you be treated? Did you have a chance? How long would you live? Would you ever get well again?

We tried to keep these questions and thoughts away from you. But Dad and I shared our worries and questions perhaps all too obviously; sometimes we just looked at each other, and sometimes we even had to leave the hospital room for a while. The same questions may have gone through your mind too, but you still were afraid to put them into words. Or maybe you were simply too weak to face them.

During the nights, when I watched over you, I was reminded of the last two weeks of my mother's life—her unspeakable suffering, her tormenting pain, her hopeless pleading for a quick death. All that kept going through my mind. During the nights, when I was awake, I used to lean over you to observe your weak breathing. A terrible thought tormented me: Wasn't there some way I could protect you, my dearest Isabell, from this cruel fate? Fortunately I did hope for a miracle, and that helped. It's so hard to see a loved one suffer. Dad, too, thought about you during the nights, and wrote you this letter.

Bonn, November 17, 1981

My Dearest!

Before I go to bed, I would like to have a little chat with you. I hope I'll be able to sleep without your good-night kiss! If I had it, I would quietly go to sleep, but now I am wondering what you are doing, whether you are already asleep, or whether pain is keeping you awake. I am comforted knowing that Mom is with you. If I could only take some of your fever and your pain, my dear, I would do anything so that you would get well soon. May the feeling that we all love you more than we can say give you strength, my good child. As your father, I love you as the child who has given us so many good, endearing, and happy things. Get well soon so that we can have you back home again. We miss you very much!

In my mind I kiss and hug you tenderly, and I hope to dream about you. I am overwhelmed by the deep love I feel for you.

Your dad

17

A new day dawned. Today we had another talk with Dr. Töbellius. He tried to make two things clear to us. First, we had to face the truth—and the truth was cruel. Your illness was terminal. Considering your situation realistically, the aim could only be to prolong your short life—with treatments, perhaps a few weeks, at best months; without treatments, maybe a few days. Nobody was willing or able to say for sure. Secondly, we should continue to hope for a miracle and firmly believe in it. Dr. Töbellius had witnessed cases in which doctors had no explanation for the healing that took place. He told us about such cases, and this gave us courage.

We asked about the chemotherapy. He hoped for a treatment opening at Dr. Jaeger's clinic in Cologne. We begged for you to stay in the hospital in Bonn, but Dr. Töbellius remained firm. He decided that if you had any chance at all, it was at Dr. Jaeger's clinic. Dr. Töbellius also told us that you would lose your hair, that patients can be very sick during chemotherapy, and that you might need several sessions. We were shattered. What should we tell you? He promised to help us.

In the afternoon the four of us sat on your bed. Dr. Töbellius informed you of the diagnosis and the severity of your illness. Not once did he mention the word "cancer"; instead he consistently described the illness as a tumor. To your question whether it was cancer he answered quietly that cancer is a form of a tumor; you had a sarcoma.

He asked you if you wanted to be treated and explained that if nothing were done, you would die very soon. You said that you wanted to live, and so you wanted to be treated. Then he told you about the clinic in

Cologne. You begged to stay in the hospital in Bonn, but again he remained firm. He had already contacted Dr. Jaeger, and you had been assigned a bed possibly for next Monday. He comforted you by telling you about his friend, Dr. L., who, as the senior physician at Dr. Jaeger's ward, would look after you personally. The three of us still would have preferred the Bonn hospital.

What the future would hold we did not know. All three of us felt like victims. We were willing to try anything. Dr. Töbellius promised to visit you in Cologne. Using your charm, you made him promise that after the right therapy had been discovered in Cologne, you could return to Bonn for further treatment. He promised he would always have a bed for you if you would need one.

BONN, NOVEMBER 19, 1981

19

My dearest Isabell,

Today Dr. Töbellius explained your condition to all of us. How courageous and self-controlled you were in accepting it all. I am so proud of you! Your nerves are much stronger than mine—even though you are the sick one. What a great human being you are! Your mom and I worry about you very much, but we are deeply convinced that you are in the best hands and that you will be helped and healed. Now we have to focus all of our energies on getting you healthy again. We firmly believe in this, and we will do everything to make it happen.

Your dad

My dearest father,

Your letter has made me so very happy because it contains so much love.

Sometimes I wonder if I deserve all this love. But situations like this are so important. They tear open our ordinary daily patterns and show us how much we really love each other. Sometimes the trivialities of everyday life cover up our great love for each other.

I'm sorry I've been crabby to Matthias so often. I always thought he didn't like me, but now he's so kind and sweet. I realize how badly I treated him sometimes.

I'm surprised over and over how lovingly you care for me. You try to read every wish in my mind. I am also very grateful to Mom. Often I was grumpy, but she never lost her patience with me.

Christian has changed into such a dear and understanding brother, and Marie helps whenever she can.

You are all the most wonderful people!

I love you lots and lots. Thank you for loving me. When I visited Lou, I realized how much I missed this love.

A thousand kisses, your daughter—who loves you, who loves you so much.

Hans Zachert

I just read your delightful and meaningful letter. I was moved and grateful for your precious words. I realized that perhaps we can say things more honestly in a letter than in *talking to one another. In a letter we can better express our feelings. I will write to you often, and I will try to be as close to you as possible, my dear child. Our hearts have always reached out to you, not only now that you are in the hospital. To us parents it was always obvious that you were entrusted to us as a most enchanting and most lovable child. Usually, parents don't say this to their children, but in times of worry and danger this knowledge should give you strength and make you happy. If you were able to look into my heart, you would see that you and your mother have a very special place (the boys too, but my love for them is somewhat different).*

My child, I love you with an unending love. We are praying for God's help in your recovery. I hug and kiss you most dearly and tenderly.

Your dad

*O*n the rest of your days in the Bonn hospital you had many visitors. On Saturday we received permission to wash your hair again. So far we didn't dare tell you that you would lose it. On Sunday, my brother Siegfried came and again took a whole series of photos: photos of Belli with a wild mane, with a shock of hair, with flowing hair, with your head slightly tilted in a coquettish look.

Then you had an idea. You were troubled because you hadn't done any Christmas shopping—even though Christmas was only five weeks away. We got the idea of sending out a family portrait. Christian and Matthias liked this idea too, so the 'lightning storm' of camera flashes continued. This was how we spent the last Sunday in the Bonn hospital. Although we were all tense, nobody wanted to say anything sad or irritating or touchy.

On Monday morning an ambulance came, and two young men drove us to the clinic in Cologne. This was a terrible drive because you were sick, and we had to stop on the freeway so you could throw up. This happened even before you had any chemotherapy.

When we arrived in Cologne on November 23, the first thing we had to do was to wait. You were assigned a bed in a room with an older woman. Dr. Jaeger was abroad to attend a seminar and was scheduled to return later in the week. The doctor on duty was an unimpressive young man—I forgot his name—with a black beard. (You know who I mean.) He said stupid things like: "We all have to die sometime, and nobody knows exactly when." But you knew how to take care of him. Dr. L. arrived in the afternoon. He was the first ray of light in Cologne: a fatherly, capable doctor. It was too soon to start treatments. He had to wait for Dr. Jaeger, and several examinations were still necessary.

A computerized tomography was planned for the following day. Your father came after work to see you. We were disappointed that we couldn't spend the night with you, but we couldn't get a private room. It was an old, small ward, not up to today's standards. After the modern, friendly hospital in Bonn, knowing we'd have to live in this ward for weeks was a big shock. The nurses seemed hardened after years of caring only for cancer patients, and their energies seemed almost depleted. They tried their best, but sometimes scars form a callous on your soul because you couldn't survive otherwise.

Then it's nearly impossible to remain sensitive and happy. We went home that evening with heavy hearts.

When I returned to Cologne the next morning, you were already in the main building for the computerized tomography. Your bed was empty, but I found an envelope addressed "To the Zachert parents."

NOVEMBER 24, 1981

My very dear parents,

I had so much to say to you, but then I was distracted. I fell asleep again because the sleeping pill was still affecting me.

Now that you cannot be near me every moment, I feel so abandoned and alone, so small and sick. I feel how important you still are for me, how much I need you, and how much I miss you in all this confusion.

Here, where I am much closer to getting well, I'm afraid I'm losing you. To them I'm just another patient, but not to you.

In love forever,

Belli

23

*D*uring the week in Cologne your lungs started to fill with fluid again. Each day it became harder for you to talk. You were given oxygen again. In these days I read *The Little Prince* by Saint-Exupéry to you—quite often with a trembling heart.

Dr. Jaeger returned Thursday, a doctor with a great

personality and a wealth of experience. When the two of you met, you immediately had great respect for one another. To you he was the person you hoped would perform a miracle. To him you became an extraordinary patient, and even more as time went on. As controlled as he was, I sometimes had the impression that he looked on you as his granddaughter.

He explained to us that he still had learned nothing about the structure of your tumor. The analysis of the tissue sample would take several weeks. In your case that was too long to wait. He had to be like a hunter who has to aim into the woods in darkness and still hit the target. He decided to try the HOK therapy, a form of chemotherapy named after Dr. Hans Otto Klein. On Thursday they inserted a subclavian catheter. This must have been a terrible night for you. A severe fever made your whole body shake. Your fear of the unknown, your questions, your pain and misery—all became so overbearing that you asked for the doctor on call that night.

I don't know what he told you, but the next day I saw the damage he had done. He confronted you with all the facts, for example, that you would lose your hair. Then it became clear to me that we had made a serious mistake in not telling you about it ourselves. But we don't always have courage when we need it. Courage has to grow from within.

Friday the chemotherapy started. You endured it splendidly. By now you also had a private room in which one of us could spend the night with you.

Dad arrived Sunday noon with Matthias and Christian. You enjoyed so much having the five of us together. Christian, then a trainee in a sporting goods store, brought you four or five training suits to choose from. You thought this was very nice of him. What made us most happy was that your lungs recovered so well after only two days of therapy. The day before, the oxygen supply had already been turned off. From that day on, you could speak loudly and clearly, and you insisted on reading a book out loud. Never before in my life had I experienced such joy. I was drenched in sweat.

In the afternoon Dad and I had a "changeover"; that's what we called it whenever we took turns staying with you. I took the boys to Aunt Eva and her husband. We were invited together with Grandma to celebrate the first Sunday in Advent. On that day I carried all the world's hope in my heart.

We soon learned how important it was to be with you during chemotherapy and how this also contributed to its success. We tried to calm your fears by being with you and, whenever possible, directing your thoughts toward pleasant and encouraging things. Whenever it was possible to bring you some joy, we tried to do it.

The chemotherapy took eight days, and it was a complete success. Now we had to start getting organized. How should we best manage our time? Your father and I wanted to make sure that one of us would always be with you. I was working half-days, while Dad had to work full-time. So I had the advantage of being more flexible with time.

I considered quitting my job, but you firmly rejected that idea. You wanted our lives to continue as normally as possible. You also knew how important my job was to me. You felt that any drastic change in our lifestyle would be unsettling.

Meanwhile a group of friends gathered around us to help. Their assistance in the small problems of life helped us cope with our big problem. It started when friends lent their second car to us; that enabled us to do our changeovers in a more flexible and less time-consuming way. Another example was our neighbor, Frau Braun, who took the laundry down from the drying room and brought it back ironed. Inge, a friend of ours and the mother of your best friend, Maren, was happy to visit you, with Maren, a paraplegic, sitting by your side in her wheelchair. You and Maren had been friends since you were five and were in the same class at the Amos Comenius School. Maren had become seriously ill when she was eight.

DECEMBER 5, 1981

My dear Maren!

Your letters always give me so much strength. Thank you for writing them. I also like your poem. I'll put in on the wall.

Your Advent calendar makes me happy, especially the little hedgehog and the round locket.

I'm so happy that my music teacher, Frau Bell, wrote to me. Please tell her that I was very glad to get her letter and that it gave me courage. She has gone through a lot of trouble.

I think that you, more than anyone else, understand how I feel on the hardest days. That's why you give me so much strength.

Yesterday I heard by phone that you are not doing so well. I and someone else are thinking a lot about you.

My dear Maren, you're like a sister to me. Hugs and kisses.

Belli

Whenever Inge had a few hours for you, she let us know ahead of time so that I could go back to my job for a while. Inge helped solve the problem about your hair. After five to six days of chemotherapy, you had only a few patches of hair, and it was too tangled for combing. Should it all be cut off? We couldn't even talk about that. I brought your red beret from home, which we used to cover your remaining hair. You said that with your yellow pajamas and red beret, you would look like a parrot. Inge couldn't stand all this. So she suggested cutting off all your hair. And fortunately this was done.

Your grandma was also a great support. At the age of seventy-four, she used public transportation to come from Bonn to Cologne to fill in the morning gap at the hospital. I was never so much aware of the value of the extended family and the importance of friends.

I'm glad that we were mistaken about only one family who had been friends. They did not show any real sympathy throughout all that time, even though they had experienced so many good things by knowing you. This, however, was our only disappointment.

After one week you were done with the first round of therapy. We all looked forward to the results of the subsequent examination. The computerized tomography revealed that the tumor was considerably smaller. Dr. Jaeger said they had made the right decision in choosing this therapy.

Now we had to get through the leukopenia, a period in which your white-blood-cell count was very low. Your immune system was shattered, and any bacteria could do you in.

To prevent the danger of infection, we had to go into isolation with you. We were not supposed to leave the room at all or only with a special gown and a mask. Visitors, too, were allowed to see you only with sterilized gowns and masks. This was a lot of trouble, but we tried to find something good about this time. I found some nice books for you and for me. In this phase of leukopenia you read *Gone with the Wind,* and later all the volumes of *Angélique.* I read *Michelangelo* and *Vincent van Gogh.* The boys recorded the most beautiful tapes for us, and soon we even had a TV. Later on Christian and Matthias could also stay with you during the leukopenia phase. They sometimes spent their weekends or school-breaks there. Even in this restrictive environment we tried to enjoy every possible diversion and pleasant experience to the fullest.

Christmas was the major theme during your first leukopenia phase. You wanted to do something to please everyone. You knitted caps and wrote letters. You even wrote a letter to your former classmates, which your teacher read aloud to all of them. Unfortunately this letter is lost, but I remember what you said. You told them that your illness made you aware of the great privilege of learning and how thankful you were. If I had been the teacher, I would have kept the letter and framed it.

I do still have the letter you wrote to Ines.

DECEMBER *12, 1981*

Dear Ines,

I want to wish you and your family a blessed and beautiful Christmas. I hope the new year will bring many good things to all of you.

This past year seems to have brought me much bad luck. As bad as it was, I would not have missed this time because I had so many good talks with my parents. I am also more content, and I appreciate the value of good health.

During this time I have received so much love—I can hardly believe it.

In ordinary life we were all so busy, but when I got sick, suddenly everyone had time for me.

All this concern for me makes me very happy and gives me strength and courage. I already have ideas about where our family can best spend our vacation so I can get completely well again and my parents can rest up.

My dear Ines, I wish you all the best. Many greetings and kisses to all of you.

Isabell

You found out about a Christmas party that was being planned for the nurses and doctors on the ward. I bought a little bottle of champagne for each one. We wrapped them like medicine bottles from the pharmacy. We hung a little card in the form of a prescription, so each one would know what you had prescribed for them. For one person you prescribed something to cure his restlessness; for another something to raise his self-confidence. For Dr. Jaeger you prescribed gunpowder so he could make a direct hit on the tumor cells. All your ideas were very funny, and the next day we heard about the joy and happiness you had given. After a short time you were the darling of the ward.

On December 18 I was allowed to take you home. The streets and even the freeways were slick because of bad winter weather. Your father was in Wiesbaden to attend a committee meeting. I had promised you and Dad that I would pick you up with our car after work, but under these wintery conditions that would have been irresponsible. Feeling desperate, I asked a friend for help. He sent me a heavier car with a driver. This car had a good heater and a telephone. We arrived three hours later than planned, and you were quite upset. After all, these were three hours of the rest of your life, three hours of your most precious time, a time of freedom, without pain, time in which you experienced the highest quality of life.

When we left Cologne, we were given a prescription as well as the schedule for your next chemotherapy session. It was planned for December 28, 1981. We had nine precious days, and that during the Christmas holidays.

We tried to make the most of every day. First you had to learn to like yourself again. It was still hard for you to look in the mirror. The therapy left just patches of hair on your head, and we had trimmed it in a very amateurish way. You could not accept yourself like that. I asked my hairdresser to visit us, and dear old Herr Beckermeyer came personally to trim your remaining hair down to a peach fuzz. Now we could at least admire the beautiful shape of your head. The peach fuzz suited you very well, and your expressive eyes were even more noticeable. We should have cut your hair before the chemotherapy began.

The Christmas holidays had to be planned and prepared in a short time. Friends brought a tree for us, and each day we received more and more presents for you and for us. Several special friends did our Christmas baking. Many people expressed how glad they were that you could stay home for a few days.

In the confusion of those weeks, Dad and I had completely forgotten our twentieth wedding anniversary on December 22. (You know how we love to celebrate the important special days in our life.) Just as I was passing the Maternus Wine House, I remembered our anniversary. It was December 22, eleven o'clock a.m. I thought: "This can't be true. For twenty years I've been married to the same man, and I forgot all about it!" I went to see Frau Maternus right away and asked her whether she would have a private room available for that evening and whether a waiter without a cough or a cold could serve us (your leukocyte count was still very low). She had a room! We quickly discussed the menu. After telling her about the circumstances, I hurried home. By now it was noon. At eight o'clock that evening I would be giving a party at the Maternus Wine House, and I hadn't even invited the guests.

You were immediately thrilled. Your dad was in Wiesbaden during the day, and he planned to return to Bonn at eight in the evening after the office Christmas party. We wanted to surprise him. Christian, Matthias, and Marie would definitely be there. Aunt Brigitte and

Grandma, and our friends Inge and Hans-Jürgen, Hajo and Loew—all from Bonn—immediately agreed to come. Siegfried and Ulli from Mannheim as well as Lou and Albert, our friends from Antwerp, started out right after I called them, in spite of snow and icy roads.

I left a message in Wiesbaden for Dad to go to the Maternus Wine House instead of coming home.

At half past seven the party began. You had the seat of honor, and you could pick your dinner partners. You chose Hajo and Hans-Jürgen. I understood you very well. Unfortunately Loew could not be there, because she was afraid that you might catch her cold. She did give you a very pretty little garnet ring, which Hajo brought for you; I still wear it today.

There was already a festive mood when Dad arrived at eight o'clock. He was completely overwhelmed. At that moment he realized that today was our wedding anniversary, and he was very happy about the party. That evening we celebrated our gratitude for many things. By ten o'clock you were exhausted, so we drove back home.

This party may have cost you a lot of energy, but it gave you at least as much inner strength. We were all very happy.

We wanted to go to church on Christmas Eve, and you insisted that we go. Our relationship to our old congregation had cooled off a little after your confirmation pastor moved; we did not all make friends with the new pastor. Matthias, with some of his classmates, had registered in another church for their confirmation classes. There we attended the family celebration of Christmas Eve with our sons. We were asked to write down our wishes on a piece of paper in the shape of a red star. We

all had the same wish: "That Belli may get well again!"
When we arrived back home, it was time for the presents. Everything was supposed to be as just like in the
old days. Dad lit the candles on the Christmas tree, and
we tried to sing: "Oh, how joyfully."

If only we hadn't done that! The candles consumed
oxygen you badly needed, and the attempt at singing
destroyed our cheerfulness. Tears ran from our eyes. It
was unbearable. Someone flung open the balcony door
so you could breathe again. After calming down, we
opened the presents. You enjoyed most the presents you
made yourself. You knitted a white pullover for me, and
for Matthias you made a tennis vest that he still wears.

For hours we were busy unpacking the presents and
reading all the wonderful letters. People we had lost contact with gave encouragement and joy to all of us. In
spite of the initial emotional disaster, it was a blessed
Christmas.

On the second Christmas day the two boys left for
the Black Forest. They went to Altglashütten to visit the
Beck family. For the last fourteen years we had rented a
Christmas vacation apartment from them. Over the years
Gerda and Ernst, the hostess and host, became our
friends. Gerda called us before Christmas to invite the
boys to visit whenever they wanted to. Now was the
time, and Gerda's offer was a godsend. We had to be back
at the clinic in Cologne on December 28. New Year's Eve
would have been very hard for us, knowing that the boys
were left at home and you were in the clinic.

Although we knew we had to focus all our energies,
time, and love on you, we were aware that Christian and
especially Matthias also needed us in this difficult time.

Matthias was only fourteen and Christian nineteen. Recently they had been left almost completely to themselves. Theresa, my maid from Portugal, did her best for them in her kind and generous way, but she could not replace a father and mother. Now the boys were going to be with Gerda, who had a big heart. And Christian and Matthias would get to see their friends there.

One little episode will show the many dangers lurking in such times of emotional strain. That year there was much snow, especially in the Black Forest. Friends picked up the boys from the train station. Christian stepped onto the platform, where he was hugged and welcomed. But where was Matthias? A few seconds before he had been in the train compartment. They looked and called out to him, even inside the train. Then the train started to move. After it pulled out of the station, Matthias appeared on the other side of the tracks. He was stuck in a snowdrift with his suitcase. He had exited on the wrong side of the train. Everyone laughed, but this carelessness could have had serious consequences.

On December 28 we went back to the hospital in Cologne. By this time we were regarded as "regulars." Everyone knew us and greeted us warmly. We had no idea that on a cancer ward everyone would grow closer with each chemotherapy session and become a true community. We wondered, hadn't we seen this young woman back in November? She always had a scarf wrapped around her head so skillfully. And what about the old lady with the thick white hair? We will have to ask Basti, the Spanish cleaning lady who is the heart of the ward.

We got "our" old room, which had become almost

like a home. This time we brought a TV and your flute. I
officially took time off from work; that allowed me to
stay with you without being rushed and without having
a bad conscience about the boys. On December 29 the
subclavian vein catheter was inserted, and the chemotherapy continued on the 30th. I vividly remember
them inserting this catheter. We rode to the main building in a hospital bus; that went well. The insertion of
the vein catheter in the neck is not a very simple procedure. Each time it was done by another doctor on duty
whom we did not know. This young doctor wanted me
to leave, but in our case he met his match, because both
of us insisted that I stay. Afterwards he was very grateful. I was able to be something that an impersonal, huge
clinic could not offer: a trusted person assisting the doctor. (Why don't hospitals make more use of mothers?)
The catheter was inserted, and you were supposed to get
up and hold the bottle out of which fluid dripped into
the catheter over your head. You had to use your own
arm as a catheter stand. That enabled us to take the hospital shuttle back to the ward.

Half an hour after the insertion, you were back in
your bed. I was very depressed, but I hoped you didn't
notice.

Chemotherapy is supposed to enhance the quality
of life, but often it is forgotten that many patients under
therapy can only count on weeks or months to live.
Their quality of life is determined not only by the degree
of pain and discomfort, but also by the daily hospital
routine and particularly by the humanity and dignity
with which they are treated. The patients' freedom and
their mobility is the third factor.

On December 31 your father joined us. The three of us wanted to be together for New Year's Eve. Because we had only two beds, one of us had to go home, but neither wanted to. I don't remember how we solved the problem. I do know that we spent the last hours of the year very happily together. First we played cards, which was a lot of fun. Psychologically, your dad was in a dilemma. Normally he tries to win every hand, but this time he wanted you to win, so you would be happy. This led him to make the strangest moves in the card game. Because I'm usually indecisive and unwilling to take chances in card games, it was not hard for me to lose.

We organized something special for our New Year's Eve meal. We invited the nurse who was on night duty. I'm glad you didn't complain about our arrangements. At midnight we watched the fireworks. Before that we laughed over the television movie, *Dinner for One*.

The new year began. We asked the same question most people ask at the turn of the year: What would it have in store for us? For us, however, the two possibilities were very different: would you experience a turn for the better, or would the new year bring the end for you?

On January 6 you did well with the second series of the chemotherapy. This time we already knew that the days after therapy would be the ones on which you had the least pain. And you wanted to be in control of those days. First you tried to persuade Dr. L. that you could just as well be at home. There fewer people would have a cold or a cough. At the hospital Basti would even enter the room with her dust cloth.

At last the doctor gave up. He yielded more to your charm than to your arguments. The first hurdle was passed. Now you had to convince Dr. Jaeger. That was much more difficult, but you managed that too, using your big brown eyes. After only five days of leukopenia, you were allowed to go home. Before that you received a few transfusions so your blood would regenerate more quickly. You had to promise Dr. Jaeger not to receive any visitors for the first few days.

We could see that you were improving. You felt much better physically, and you looked forward to taking charge of your life for the next twenty-one days at home. As your white-blood-cell count went up, your friends were allowed to visit you. Before that we planned to buy you a wig. A lady hairdresser came to show you a selection: long, short, with and without a ponytail. But each wig looked worse than the other, and not even the nicest wig could replace your own hair. You decided to wear hats and berets instead. That way only a few short wisps of your hair would show, and you could stand that.

Then you were ready for your friends. And they came—even Maren in her wheelchair. What a commitment that was for her parents—and what a great help Maren was to you! She showed you how to accept your destiny and to learn to be happy with the rest of your life. She had already coped with her destiny for seven years, and she was ahead of you in maturity, enduring suffering, and life management. At this time she was a great role model for you, and she gave you much strength. You started to think that happiness might be possible even without playing tennis.

As a family we were much relieved in these days. This break between therapies was the most relaxing one.

We were certain that from now on you would only get better.

Daily life continued in a relatively normal fashion. Dad went to his office, Christian worked at the store, Matthias and Marie went to school, and I went to my office. Theresa, our Portuguese maid, came over every morning. I usually left home before eight o'clock, and I was glad to work a few hours overtime. You usually slept until ten o'clock. Then you took a bath; sometimes Grandma stopped by or one of my friends. You often called me at my office at around eleven to make plans for the afternoon. It was a great help to me that my job was less than half a mile from home. That gave me the security of knowing that I could always be with you in a few moments. This was comforting for you too. When I would get home at noon, meals and housekeeping were done, and we were free to enjoy the afternoon and the evening.

We even went shopping downtown in the last days before your third series of chemotherapy. You enjoyed that so much. You especially appreciated little things: a pretty tin container with tea, a small silver ring, a beach bag for summer. You were not so much interested in real necessities but looked for small luxuries. For you the ring was the symbol of a present you dreamed of, which you would receive later in your life. The pretty little tea container would be part of your dowry, and the beach bag allowed you to dream about the Caribbean.

Never before had I experienced so much joy in shopping. I was grateful that we had the financial means to do that. Many parents of cancer patients can barely manage to buy the necessities—and often not even that.

The beautiful days at home came to an end. You had to be back in Cologne Monday, February 1, 1982. On Sunday we wanted to have one more big celebration. All of us wanted to spend that day with the von Moltke family. We had known their children since elementary school. Both you and Johannes attended the same class at the Amos Comenius School. The twins, Dorothea and Daniel, were the same age as Matthias. The two boys were good friends, and that was a gift to us parents. We had noticed how lonely Matthias was at this time, and we could offer hardly any help. The von Moltkes took him in. Ulrike and Konrad, the parents, told him that he would always have a home with them. They not only handed him the house keys as a symbol, but made him welcome at all times.

We met with them for brunch at the club and celebrated this Sunday. They also brought along their fourth child, Jacob—a little latecomer. It was a casual, relaxed Sunday with no depressing thoughts.

On February 1 we went back to Cologne. For the past few days you had pain in your left foot. Was this perhaps connected to the operation you had last year? Or due to the pins that still remained in the ankle? Or was it cancerous growths? A scintigraphy of the bone was made. The doctors could not agree about the result. There may have been something visible; on the other hand they hoped that your pain was caused by the pins. It was decided to remove the pins after two more chemotherapy treatments. The doctors' explanations were a bit vague. It was not like you to accept this, but we all were so concentrated on overcoming your illness that we didn't want to think about this new problem.

In the HOK therapy, the fourth day is a day of rest. It happened to be a Saturday. You took advantage of Dr. L.'s visit to ask him if you could spend that day at home. I was aware of the heavy responsibility and the possible consequences for the doctors who would permit something like that; they were not supposed to allow a home visit. On the other hand, we all knew that a few hours at home—hours of normality—would do more good than the therapy. A few days at home would also be good for your balance. The days of painful chemotherapy would be offset by the days of living without pain, days of being free. And each day that was worth living increased your willingness to endure the next series of treatments. Fortunately Doctor L. understood this and allowed us to go home. (I wonder why hospitals can't allow doctors to be more flexible in making such decisions with critically ill patients.)

During these days of therapy, you were often depressed and desperate. It bothered you that the lives of all of us were restricted by your illness. I still remember one conversation in which you talked about your illness as a burden on our lives. I tried to explain that I didn't feel it as a burden but as a chance to have a particularly close relationship to you. Never before was my life filled with such deep meaning. By my mere presence, I was able to take away or at least alleviate the fear of another human being.

Your question was perhaps caused by the casual remark of a doctor who was on duty one Saturday. In the morning he saw us together in your room and then again in the evening. Surprised, he asked us: "What, you're still here?"

"I live here with my daughter while she is in therapy,"
I replied. "I'm on vacation here!"

"What, you're on vacation here in the hospital?" he
said. He was amazed, but he showed respect. I had taken
ten days of vacation from work. Considering the circumstances, it was a wonderful time for me. Without being
rushed, I was able to dedicate myself to you completely.
I sensed how valuable this was for you, and that made
me very happy.

You also met Dr. P. during this series of treatments.
She was the senior physician at the Cologne Children's
Clinic, and we had known her for ten years. When I was
in despair, I would talk with her. She was able to give me
much support by sharing her thoughts, and even more
by listening well to me. From her I learned that it is possible to live with thoughts about death and that sup-
pressing such thoughts is of no help to a critically ill
person. Furthermore she told me that people are willing
to fight differently when they know about the seriousness and the finality of the struggle. Most important,
she also taught me how to let go of a loved one so that
the person can die in peace.

I knew that I had to take advantage of every minute
with you. The fulfillment of our destiny did not lie in
prolonging your life, but in how we would make use of
this period of life together, given to us by God.

You were happy each time Dr. P. visited you. The two
of you developed a relationship of great trust, and you
became very good friends.

At the beginning of February, Matthias wrote a letter
to you that must have made you very happy.

Dear Sister!

*I don't know where I should begin. Let me start with
where I met you for the first time. This was, I think, in my
baby bed. You always were, and you still are, very lively. You
jumped and bounced around everywhere. Your enormous
charm was unstoppable.*

*Time passed and we grew older. You always stood at my
side, as you always will, and you supported me whenever
you could. I was so young that I didn't even notice it. When
I started to grow, just as you did, we found out that we both
had power, just like today. We also found out that this
power could be used to make each other angry, but I know
that this was all in fun because we always loved and still
love each other so much.*

*Years went by. From acting like a boy you changed into a
cute girl. A new phase began. I think I was afraid to lose a
good playmate from the sandbox. That's why I called you
names. I teased you about being a person who would use
makeup and who wouldn't associate with small children still
playing in the sandbox. And I was hurt whenever Dad would
give you a bigger hug (which he will always do). I believe that
this was only jealousy because I too wanted to have a little
love from this blossoming young girl—and I still do.*

*Time did not stand still. Both of us grew older, and the
time came when you went to kindergarten. I was not yet
allowed to go. It must have been a hard time for me because
I didn't get to see you until noon when kindergarten was
over. I always waited at the window and watched for you.
Finally I saw your little head turn toward me with a bright
smile—like the beams of a rising sun, which is fascinating
over and over again.*

I was glad when I finally was able to go to kindergarten too. I hung onto your skirt as well as to your hand. You led me to my other playmates, who were there too. At the time I thought that you didn't want me anymore, but that was not true. You only wanted to show me that I couldn't always be with you and that I should have other playmates as well. That helped me a lot.

Then came the time when you didn't have to go to kindergarten anymore. You were ready for elementary school. I was still so little—a small, foolish, unimportant thing in this world. After I also finished my time in kindergarten, I went to elementary school too. I was glad you were there to welcome me. By this time you had advanced to second grade, and with your smile you had won a whole host of friends. They always stood at my side whenever I had a quarrel with classmates.

This beautiful time passed by as well. You went to high school, the school for big kids. I still stayed in elementary school, the school for little ones. Even then I had trouble getting along with others.

Time went by and I went to high school as well. Again, I felt protected.

Just as you took me to school and to kindergarten, you also brought me to the tennis club. There they all knew me because they knew the girl with the bright smile. You introduced me there as well.

What I am trying to say, or better yet, what I mean, is that you are like a support made out of diamonds—the hardest stone of all—on which I can really depend.

Dear Isabell, my sister, I want to tell you that I love you forever, that my love is always with you, especially in difficult times. A flower wilts when it does not get any sunlight.

I'm such a flower, your brother who needs your life-sustaining sunlight. I feel how my leaves are wilting.

Dear sister, I wish you well from the bottom of my heart, because we all need you, your love, and your smile. We all look forward to seeing you come back home again. Your brother who loves you,

"The Baby"

P.S. You don't need to write back. Don't waste your energies. I know that you love me, just as I love you from the bottom of my heart. We wish you all the best!

On February 15 we were allowed to go home, this time for a four-week break.

I took Matthias to the hospital February 16 because of a comparatively small problem. His nasal cavities and sinuses were frequently congested, and he always had colds. During your leukopenia he was not allowed to have any contact with you, because we were afraid you might catch a bacterial infection. So he had to live with the von Moltke family.

We decided we had to change that. Dr. Maurer recommended operating on his nasal septum. This was a relatively simple procedure, but with all the family pressures, it was extremely hard for Matthias. I was unable to care for him the way he wanted. He had hoped to receive an extra portion of love, care, and sympathy. Fortunately he was able to get over his disappointment.

When Matthias was released from the hospital, we focused all our thoughts on your sixteenth birthday, which was on March 3, 1982. We wanted to have a big celebration with all our friends. However, the big party could not be too strenuous for you. We counted all the friends and ended up with twenty-four people. We invited them all to the club, where we felt at home.

First of all, the party needed to be organized. Naturally you were involved. You were in charge of the seating arrangement and the place cards. You wanted Albert and Siegfried to be your dinner partners. They were definitely the most lively characters. You made the place cards yourself: on the outside the person's name and a picture, on the inside a few special words for each one. We wondered, would they all come?

Everyone came! Even Lou and Albert came with Caroline and Axel from Antwerp, Ines from Munich, Siegfried and Ulli from Mannheim—they all took a day off work. According to the medical prognosis, this would be your last birthday, but nobody wanted to accept that. They all did their best to make this celebration an unforgettable experience for you. While we were afraid that this might be your last birthday party, we were happy to celebrate it with you. For a long time afterwards we drew strength from that party, and its memories still make me happy.

The weekend following your birthday we drove with you to Belgium to visit Lou and Albert for the first time. That shows how well you were again, how joy and happiness had returned to your life. Christian and Matthias came along. You looked forward to seeing Lou and Caroline, but you especially wanted to see Axel. His eyes were just as beautifully brown as yours. The two of you conversed only with glances, but it was obvious that you were fascinated by each other. (Axel is now a very successful, self-employed landscape architect. Albert died last year; he had a heart attack while playing tennis, but you know that better than I.)

On this weekend, Lou planned to celebrate Axel's birthday. You were fully involved in the celebration. Naturally the birthday cake was for both of you. Lou did everything to make this weekend enjoyable for us. Whenever we were in Belgium, we had a good time. Lou even came to Cologne and Bonn, sometimes only for a few hours, just to bring joy and a little diversion. The whole family loved you, and your relationship to Caroline and to Axel was a third-generation friendship. My parents and Lou's had been friends first. How good it is to reap fruit in one's own lifetime!

MARCH 9, 1982

Hello my Angel Doris!

I get to do more and more things. I celebrated my birthday with a real bang. I made my first trip to Belgium. I will go to school for one hour on Thursday. And today I will go shopping in Bonn. Not bad, don't you think? Perhaps I will visit the ninth-graders, because I know I couldn't keep up in my old class.

Ingund and Anton are in the ninth grade, and the teachers are very good too. Frau Keller is the class teacher.

You know what I saw? Yesterday I went to my tennis club to visit my old team. They all acted a bit odd, as if they didn't know how to treat me.

*I've noticed this already with several people. Many have
also told me that I've changed. My uncle said that I wasn't
as cheerful and funny as I used to be, but I haven't felt that
at all. I find such behavior toward me strange and not very
nice. Hopefully that will end soon. In general I hope that
everything will become normal again, because my parents
are at the end of their rope.*

*Dear Doris, I wish you all the best. Greetings to
your parents.*

Belli

Before we returned to Cologne, you insisted on
going back to school once more. You were so
excited about that—but you came back so disappointed. You wanted, above all, to surprise the class,
but neither the students nor the teachers were prepared.
You dressed up very elegantly—quite sassy with a beret
and sunglasses and a stylish scarf around your neck. You
did not look like a person who is critically ill. Your classmates were confused. They didn't dare look at you
because they wanted to avoid staring at your wig. Was it
really a wig? You looked so stylish, and no one wanted
to stare.

No one knew what to say. Everyone had a thousand questions, like, "Is it true that you have cancer?"
"Are you dying?" But nobody broached the subject out
of fear of saying something wrong. But they didn't
want to talk about the weather or the latest test either.
That didn't seem right.

You longed so much for them to give you a hug, to tell you how happy they were to see you again, that they hoped you would continue to fight bravely, that they might visit you during your next chemotherapy session to tell you all about school, that it was amazing how great you looked. Unfortunately, we did not let the class know that you really wanted to celebrate.

On March 15, 1982, we went back to Cologne. This time Dad accompanied you to the chemotherapy session. This one was very tough. A new therapy, called DTIC, was tried. Now there were sources of information: people shared their experiences in the hallway. All the patients were so well acquainted by now that you visited one another in your rooms when circumstances allowed. We had heard that with each therapy the tumor cells would become more and more resistant. We wondered if that was the reason for changing the therapy. Dr. Jaeger calmed us down and explained that he wanted to use a second "weapon." He would save the HOK therapy for later.

DTIC, however, did not agree with you at all. Dad told me that in the nights—when you couldn't sleep— you repeatedly asked him about life after death. Together you speculated. His hypotheses were a bit more abstract, while yours were more concrete. At one time Dad's powers of imagination must have gotten low. He said that he could not picture very well life after death. If everyone would go to heaven, he said, it would have to be closed eventually because of overcrowding. This joking remark probably restored the peace of the night.

During the days, Dad tried to stimulate you to do something creative. He encouraged you to play your flute. Music had always been important for you in the past. At the age of nine you registered for piano lessons at the music school all on your own, even though we didn't have a piano. It was hard enough for parents who owned a piano to find lessons for their talented children, but you managed it anyway. After all, you said, you could always practice at a friend's home. We had no other choice but to buy a piano. For the first and only time in our life, we had to start time payments in order to buy it. You became quite good at playing the piano, and you also played the flute.

Now you began to think about music again and wanted to play your flute. Like the Pied Piper of Hamelin you attracted visitors into your hospital room. These sounds were so unusual in the ward that everyone, including Basti and Dr. Jaeger, wanted to know where they came from. In these moments you were able to completely forget everything. One of your favorite pieces was a song with the words, "The devil can do many, many things. But he cannot sing." When one of us was about to leave and stood at the door, you would say: "Wait, let me just play the sad 'note.'" You held this note for a long time until it grew weaker and weaker. Then you often had a tear in your eye, and whenever you were in a good mood, you gave us that tear as a farewell. You would take it with your finger from your cheek and lay it on my mouth.

You also started to paint again and completed the beautiful picture with the pastel-colored hollyhocks. Friends had brought you these flowers and Dad encouraged you to paint them. Dr. P. has written a paper on the meaningfulness of pictures drawn by children with tumors. You will be happy to know that your pictures are among the drawings analyzed. Shortly before the outbreak of your illness you made a collage. Dr. P. thought this picture had a particularly intense aura and gave a strong message. Even a television documentary has been made about your picture—but I'm sure you know this.

After this therapy session you had to remain in strict isolation in the hospital for sixteen days. Your blood profile was disastrous. The examination results, however, were promising. We were relieved, and we asked Dr. Jaeger for a detailed report on the continuation of the treatment. You knew about this talk and you wanted to come along, but he invited only us parents to his office. He congratulated us on the achievements of the chemotherapy and pointed out that the therapy accounted for only half the success. The other half was due to our commitment. However, he said, everything done so far was only the beginning. If you had a chance to get well at all, we would have to persevere for two or three years.

Although this was fairly good news, we felt as if the bottom had fallen out. How could we possibly hang on for two or three more years? We were entirely unprepared for this message. For the second time it was like being stabbed by a sword!

What were we supposed to tell you? An hour ago we thought that in half a year we would have accomplished everything! Again we stood in front of your door, crying, not knowing how to proceed. This time Dr. Töbellius was not there; there was no one who could help us talk to you. We tried to tell you gently. The thought of being tied to this kind of life in the hospital for two or three more years was unbearable for you. We began to sense, too, that our energies would not hold out for such a long time. If only it were possible to continue the treatments in Bonn. We had other children who needed us. We had used up our vacation days, and leaving you alone in Cologne during chemotherapy was unthinkable. Contacts with your school, your class, and your friends were also very important to you, and the clinic in Cologne was quite a distance for students from Bonn.

You planned to say all this to Dr. Jaeger during his next visit. When he came, Dr. L., Dad, and I were there too. "I have to talk to you. Do you have time for me?" you asked. Dr. Jaeger sat on your bed. This was the first time he had done this, and it was quite unusual for this distinguished gentleman. You sat upright in your bed. Without saying a word, you and he looked into each other's eyes for a long time. The silence created tension in the room. Dr. Jaeger was ready to listen, and you concentrated on your choice of words. "Why can't I continue the chemotherapy at the hospital in Bonn?"

"Don't you like me anymore?" he asked.

"I do, very much, like my own grandfather," you replied. "But . . . ." Then you listed all the arguments you had carefully prepared.

He listened to everything patiently, still looking straight into your eyes. When he did not answer, you flipped the tip of his nose and said: "Please!"

"The next HOK therapy in Bonn then," he agreed, "but after that back to Cologne, please."

We were so happy. Here was a ray of hope! Now we only had to wait for your leukocyte count to go back up. We wanted to spend our Easter holiday in the Black Forest.

But the leukos did not increase. The time for your release was postponed day after day. On Maundy Thursday we were finally allowed to go home. This time it was quite a move: painting utensils, books, cassettes, radio, pictures, and the TV. We had lived in the hospital four weeks.

We had hardly arrived back home when you wanted to go to Altglashütten as soon as possible, because the next chemotherapy session was scheduled to begin in ten days. That same day Dad and I packed the suitcases. In the evening we dropped off Christian. Some time ago he had registered, through his employer, for a scuba diving course in Corfu. Now he would have much preferred to go with us, but it was too late to cancel his trip. Marie went to visit her parents in Belgium, which meant that Matthias would be the only young person to be there with you. We asked the von Moltkes whether any of their children would like to come with us. Daniel and Dorothea had already left for their break, but Johannes wanted to join us by train on Easter Sunday.

What a memorable time this was! There was still enough snow in the Black Forest to cover the landscape like magic. Once again, Gerda had lovingly prepared our attic apartment in their remodeled barn. We were the only visitors, and the weather was good. Unfortunately Dad suffered from an infection of the middle ear.

You had a great longing for fresh air and for nature. I tried to take you for a few walks. Whenever you went outside, you wore Dad's fur hat, which covered all of your head. Your face was visible only from your eyes down to your chin. It looked so natural that you did not need to wear a wig underneath. When you were too warm, you even took off the hat for several minutes when nobody saw you. You didn't care about your bald little head. When we returned to our country-style living room, it became quite natural for you to run around without a wig. What would you do when Johannes arrived on Sunday? At first you were a little shy, but after Johannes said that he found you much more attractive without the wig, the ice finally broke and you went without the wig—at least inside the apartment.

In the evenings the five of us played cards or a dice game. For a few moments we managed to be completely normal, happy, and relaxed, but at times we also became touchy; our souls were wounded and our nerves on edge. We tried to cover that up and keep our balance, but we were not always able to do that.

Johannes was a great help to all of us. Matthias was happy to have a friend there who was healthy and normal and who was not always thinking in terms of cancer, chemotherapy, and fear. Johannes' presence helped us to be more careful in choosing our words and directing our thoughts—and for you it was a blessing! The two boys treated you in a completely natural, humorous, uncomplicated way. Every day they challenged you to test your physical limits. Whenever you didn't want to walk anymore, they started a snowball fight, and whenever you really couldn't walk, the boys took turns carrying you on their backs or in their arms. (I still dream about my father carrying me in his arms; he did that only once, thirty-five years ago!)

We also took a ride on a horse-drawn sleigh. You said you felt so good wrapped in blankets, exposed to the sun and the fresh air of the Black Forest. We took a break at noon, and you built a small dam in the creek next to the Raimarti Lodge. Each day you moved about with more self-confidence. Now you often took off your fur hat, but you did not yet allow us to take pictures of your shaved head. On a longer walk, Dad once tried to catch you with his camera right after you had taken off your hat. You hid behind big Johannes. He immediately understood the situation and winked at Dad. After a few seconds he winked again and moved his body a bit sideways. In that instant Dad took the picture. This was the first photo of you with your shaved head, and it is still one of our favorites. From that moment on you were not afraid to face the camera just as you were.

You became stronger, and your confidence in your body grew. Your appetite increased too. During the day we stopped at all the cozy inns we had come to know over the past fourteen years. I especially remember a hike around Lake Schluch. It was a sunny but cold day. Your physical fitness had improved so much that we dared to hike as far as the old Black Forest inn, *Unterkrummenhof,* for many years a favorite destination on our hikes. A recent snowfall covered the landscape with enchantment. So much zest for life made you almost giddy. The fields of snow excited you, and you wanted to go sledding. We didn't have a sled with us, but we had a plastic bag. We made do with it to slide down every slope that was still covered with snow. When we arrived at the *Unterkrummenhof,* you hung up your wet coats by the tiled stove, and then the three of you snugly warmed up on the tiled bench connected to the stove. Suddenly you were ready: inside the inn you took off your hat, and you didn't care about the people staring at you.

Naturally, we ate a hearty meal, and you tried to keep up with the boys. If it hadn't been for the appointment with the doctor to check your leukocyte count, we would almost have completely forgotten your illness.

On Sunday we drove home because we had to be in the Bonn hospital on Monday. You were taken to your old ward. Burbi was still there as the doctor in charge. The nurses greeted you with great joy. The same day, Dr. Töbellius inserted a catheter. This time you did not have to take the shuttle to another building to see a strange doctor and then return on foot. It was so much easier staying here! Dr. Töbellius came into your room and inserted the catheter himself, and you had no fear because you had great confidence in him.

We had always thought that Dr. Töbellius must have a wife and many children. How else was he able to sympathize so well with us? We had never asked him about his family, but now we learned from a talkative patient in the hallway that he was a bachelor. The reason for that soon became clear to us: he was, in a sense, married to the hospital and to his patients. He was always there, and he did everything for his patients—as you so often experienced.

I only need to think about your "Why" picture. In the Bonn hospital you started to draw the faces of your visitors, and—using a mirror—you also drew your own face with a pencil. You finished it in a short time, and it was remarkable. The expression of fear, and the piercing question "Why?" lay in your eyes. Your red lips revealed an awakening desire. You asked each visitor to react to that picture. As they looked at the picture, you asked them pointed questions. If they looked away or gave you a superficial answer, you considered them failures. If they sensed the outcry of your picture and were willing to talk to you about your fears and dreams, they passed the test. That afternoon I witnessed several such "exams," and I was put to the test myself. I also was unable to answer your question about the "Why," but together we searched for a way.

Dr. Töbellius came to visit in the afternoon and asked how you were doing. You showed him the picture and asked what he would have to say about it. "This is supposed to be you? Well, listen, you are much prettier than that. But it is a very important picture. We have to talk about it sometime when we won't be disturbed. Come to my office this evening. I'll let you know when." At around six o'clock he called you downstairs and talked with you for an hour and a half.

Afterwards you told me that you had talked about life and death and also about a very personal problem. Several days later Dr. Töbellius told me that he couldn't remember any conversation with a patient that was as intense as the one with you. That evening you wanted to write a letter to thank him for the talk. You asked me if that was appropriate.

"Why not?" I replied.

You showed the letter to me, and then the content of your conversation became partly clear to me. You apparently asked him for advice on how you should behave with Axel. Should you write to Axel and tell him about your affection for him? What if you would be rejected? Dr. Töbellius made it clear to you that life cannot be won without taking chances, and you thanked him for this insight. I don't know if this letter still exists, but in my heart I still remember it. You then told me that if you ever married, you hoped for a husband with whom you could have such good conversations.

On Sunday the confirmation of your cousin Oliver took place. My brother planned a big family reunion in Bonn. We really hoped you could be there, too, especially because they lived only a few blocks from the hospital. The rest of the family gathered in nearly perfect weather. Dad and I were with you in the hospital where you were undergoing chemotherapy. Your blood profile was still normal, so I asked Dr. Töbellius if there was any chance at all of leaving the hospital. He said yes!

What should you wear? You had so much fun deciding which hat, which wig, which glasses, which pullover—a little makeup? You wanted everyone to be delighted, and you also wanted to look good—and that was quite normal.

You had fun saying goodbye in the nurses' lounge. "The sickest patient is going out!" you cried. Quite a few other patients who were not nearly as ill as you were had to think about that.

The confirmation was wonderful, and Oliver was happy. After two hours we went back to the hospital, because you wanted to rest. We all planned to return to the party in the afternoon. However, as it often happens during chemotherapy, you experienced a severe mood swing. Excited and lively in the morning, in the afternoon you were depressed and desperate. It took all my art of persuasion and powers of motivation to get you out of your bed and out of your depression. Once you were back at the party, you were happy again. Siegfried took another beautiful series of photos.

You did not bring Oliver a present, but you wrote him a very nice letter.

Dear Oliver,

I hope that you realize the meaning of your confirmation. To many, this gets lost in all the gifts.

Today I won't give you a present, because I could not think of anything meaningful, but whenever I can help you with something, I'll gladly do it, just as you have often helped me.

Hugs and kisses,

Isabell

Each treatment made you more and more depressed. During these treatments we did not sleep with you at night because you didn't want us to.

You wanted to give us a break, and we were grateful for that. However, during the night I often felt fear in my heart. The balcony of your room was so high up—and your mood was often so low.

Just two days after the end of the treatments you were allowed to go home. We had to have your blood profile checked every other day. For you as a patient this therapy was so much better, offering so much more diversion. You could stay in your natural environment where you were close to your friends, and where you could spend the time of leukopenia at home. In case of an emergency, the Bonn hospital was much closer. Going to Cologne took us about an hour, while getting to the Bonn hospital took only ten minutes. The ratio of the painful treatment days and the days worth living improved.

Certainly some changes could be made in the treatment of children with cancer. There could be new ways that would provide more flexibility, more opportunities for treatment at home. I am sure that I could have figured out how to change an infusion bottle if someone had showed me. Why can't hospitals work together with the family doctors, the patients, and their families? Aren't there psychologists who could help families cope? In medical terms the last years have certainly led to great accomplishments in fighting cancer, but more consideration of the psychological situation of the patients and their families would greatly add to these accomplishments.

We now had a break of nine weeks ahead of us. During this time we were in a state of euphoria. Often I was afraid that the many experiences would be too much for you, but you wanted to live. Summer came, and everyone wanted to do something good for you. When you were not yet allowed to go outside, we had fun at home. Caroline came from Antwerp for a few days. You enjoyed yourselves playing tapes of music on your new stereo. You could also talk about Axel, which was very important to you.

You were able to celebrate Matthias' confirmation in May. You were not allowed inside the crowded church because of your low white-blood-cell count and the danger of catching an infection, but you did join us for the family celebration. You were very happy that the entire von Moltke family was there too.

The Communion service took place ten days later. This time you could come along. You wanted to meet Matthias' confirmation pastor. There were many people in church. Family groups were invited to the Communion, each time a group of about forty believers. The pastor passed the chalice from person to person. Dad and I weren't sure if you wanted to walk to the front of the church with us. Of course, all we could think about were the germs of all the believers jumping around in the Communion cup, and we were afraid you might catch an infection. When it was our turn, you stood, wearing your white dress and a white hat, in that large semicircle, surrounded by us. The pastor took a new, clean chalice, filled it with wine and served it to you first. God was indeed with us!

There were other diversions and pleasant events: Marie brought two big suitcases from Belgium filled with theater costumes. What a great time you had! In one afternoon you changed into many costumes and characters. We provided the necessary background music, and Marie took photos. You were a spirited Spanish lady, a seductive vampire, a cowgirl, a romantic "flower child," a rock singer, a motorcycle driver, and then back to Belli again—just as she was, completely normal, with beret, wig, and scarf.

You both enjoyed this kind of nonsense, even though Marie was twenty and you were sixteen, no longer at the age of dressing up for fun. But for you there was a chance to try on many life roles in a short time.

Marie was really a sweetheart. More and more you were like sisters. On her next visit from Belgium, she brought you a little album with all these photos.

By the end of May—as soon as you came out of the leukopenia and were allowed to leave the house—you went walking and shopping together. Often Dorothea von Moltke came along as well. I usually remained close by as an "escort" in case anything would happen.

Meanwhile you had intense pain in your arm and for one day you had to go to Cologne for another computerized tomography and a bone scintigraphy; every now and then you received outpatient treatment at the Bonn hospital. You accepted these visits—as long as you knew that you were not returning for long-term chemotherapy.

You also went to see Siegfried, Ulli, and little Sascha. Little Sascha was a great joy to you. Ulli and Siegfried had asked you to be the godparent of their daughter, which made you very happy. Not only did they trust you to care for the baby, they also gave you the assurance that they believed you would go on living. These were enchanting days for you. Ulli and Siegfried really spoiled you!

We again drove to Belgium. First you were with Marie and her parents for two days and then with Lou. Everyone grew fond of you: Robert and Rosita (Marie's parents) and her remarkable grandparents, Anne (Marie's sister), and even their housekeeper. Almost weekly Rosita sent the most delightful cards to you. These cards had images of dreams, each one more beautiful than the other, and Rosita added comments in her broken German. The days with Lou were exciting. She prepared a big party the weekend before my birthday.

My brothers, Siegfried and Rolli, and their families were also invited, along with many friends. In their big garden they had pitched a tent. We danced and laughed, talked to each other in French, English, and German, and ate and drank long into the night.

Every now and then my eyes and my heart reached out to you. You kept yourself in the background. The other children all helped with the serving, but you weren't really able to help them. Perhaps you hoped for a glance or even a conversation with Axel. But this never happened. Maybe Axel liked you too much already!

When we drove home, you were a little sad. Leaving Antwerp was hard for you. The prospect of Lou's children visiting us soon comforted you. Axel, Caroline, and Kathy—the oldest sister—arrived a few days later. They also brought Friedemann, Axel's German friend, whom you knew as well.

Axel and Friedemann wanted to clean up our vacation place in Oberwinter and stay overnight. It had been vacant for the last few months. The two girls stayed with you in your room. You really enjoyed that! Kathy was lovesick, and Caroline had just fallen in love. And you contributed by sharing your "experiences" from *Angélique*. Often the three of you talked until late into the night. The relationship with Axel did not develop any further. (I wish I could have been a little mouse in your room!)

You again made contact with your friends from the tennis club. Playing tennis was out of the question, of course. But during the Pentecost holidays your old team organized a youth tournament, and Sibylle Pagenkopf, your former tennis coach, asked you to help manage it.

What a joy it was for you to take part, to belong again. Questions were directed to you: "Miss Zachert, when can I play?" "Isabell, may I have new tennis balls, please?" "What was the score?" You were needed again, and you had something to say.

Just a few days earlier we had stood at the fence of another tennis club and watched. You had a popsicle, and you looked quite sassy. A young man stood next to us. We hadn't noticed him at first. After a while he said: "You're Isabell Zachert, aren't you? People say that you're sick, but you don't look sick!"

"The sickness I have is supposed to be terminal. Usually people die from it!" was your answer. And you probably thought, "But I won't!"

Now you were back in the middle of things. The weather played along and helped make the tournament a success. In the evening a last big party with a dance was planned at the club house. But your right arm hurt again. We had to at least ask the doctors for advice. We saw the second senior physician in the Bonn hospital during the Pentecost holidays. She liked you very much and I told her about my reservations regarding the dance. She said: "Give her an extra-strength painkiller and let her go." The star of the junior league opened the dance with you. You hadn't taken your dancing lessons, but that didn't matter. You were musical, and you knew how to move. When I picked you up at eleven p.m., you were ecstatic. You had danced all evening, this was your prom, the ball of your life. Thomas Graner later looked after you in a very dear and friendly way.

My dear Maren!

This letter will be somewhat difficult because—this could drive me crazy—my arm hurts again. I made a wrong move earlier, and now my writing is so sloppy.

Please forgive me that I did not get in touch with you in the last few days. I really couldn't write, and there was so much going on last weekend that I had no time. Our tennis club organized a youth tournament on Saturday, which was really super. Many clubs from Bonn were invited, and always their top girl and the two top-seated boys. There was much going on, and I helped in the office behind the stand. In that place some people who would otherwise have ignored me were very polite. It was wonderful to be with young people who behaved naturally because they didn't know anything about my condition.

In the evening we had a party that started very slow. Many of the club members had not arrived yet, so many curious outsiders soon left, which was quite all right. This was my first party in a year. At 9:30 the party finally got started, and guess what, I got to dance the opening dance with Thomas Graner! After we started dancing, the dance floor began to fill up immediately. Everyone had been wanting to dance, but nobody dared start. The evening before I was so sad because I didn't think I could be there. But we got stronger medicine that made it possible for me to go.

All day Sunday we were with the von Moltkes in Oberwinter. That was very nice, and I got a great tan. We were in a bad mood only once because Matthias was arguing with everyone, and in return everyone told him off, but that passed.

I can only say that the weekend was very nice.

I hope it was for you too. I'll take a break now.

Have I told you that the pins in my ankle have been removed? That wasn't the most pleasant experience in my life, but I had expected it to be different. I was so scared, because I had no idea what would happen. During the break between getting a shot and pulling the pins, they left me completely alone. That wasn't very nice, because I imagined all sorts of thoughts.

Dear Maren, I may call you tonight.

I think about you a lot.

Your Belli

P.S. Greetings from everyone.

65

At the end of May, Dad and I met Hatty and Paul Martin, a Canadian couple. Within a short time they became good friends. They had two children, Theresa and Jan. Getting to know this family was a blessing for all of us because they tried to bring joy and hope into our lives. The Martins had strong faith and natural joy in living. First we had to learn how to play Bingo at the club. We dressed up and reserved a table where there was no draft and where nobody close by was smoking. We ate, and then the game was on. We talked in English. The children sat at one end of the table, we parents at the other. Jan sat opposite you. He had many interesting things to tell you. He was three years older than you, very self-confident and determined. He didn't seem at all awkward in your presence. For you that was a new experience.

Destiny must have wanted you to win the game. You had to walk up to the stage, and those who knew you were very happy. After the game you had to go to the bathroom. That wasn't noteworthy, except that you did not return. Jan was also gone. Dad became anxious, but Hatty reassured him, "They'll come back!"

After a while Christian went out to look for you and returned very excited. "They're taking a walk in the park!" he said. For you this was the beginning of a wonderful time. The two of you fell in love. Jan came to visit you at home almost every day. First we would all visit together. You children then took Jan to Christian's or Matthias' room to talk about soccer or music. After that you and Jan went to your room. These hours were wonderful for you. Christian couldn't stand the door being closed. He always found a reason to go inside. One time he came out filled with dismay: "He's kissing her!" How happy I was!

For a long time already you had taken off your wig when Jan was there. He told you that he would see only your beautiful eyes.

Whenever Christian became too curious and jealous, I took a chair and sat at your door like a watchdog. These visits with Jan were the most beautiful hours of your day. Later you wrote a letter to Jan in English.

My Dear Jan,

The evening yesterday was lovely. It gave me very much power.

I'm very excited if you kiss me. It is such a nice feeling. You can't imagine what a great feeling it is if I know that you will like me the way I am. You know I am ill, but just for some time. When I have to stay in bed, I need nice things to think of.

I kiss you so sweet and soft.

Your Isabell

However, there were also other things for you to think about. Maren's condition had grown worse. She had to go to an orthopedic clinic in Münster for the fitting of a corset. You were very concerned about her.

You went back to school for a few hours at a time, but that did not work out well. We thought you could repeat this class after the summer break. And after considering which teachers and classmates you would have, you chose a new class that was one year below your old one.

MAY 24, 1982

Dear Maren,

Unfortunately I have to write with my left hand, because my right arm is hurting too much.

You have been in Münster already for many hours. I hope the change was not too hard for you. I promise to support you and help you however I can.

With few exceptions I find my class very dumb. I made the decision to repeat the school year in class 9a. I don't feel like part of my old class anymore; I'm like an outsider. I also feel I'm in the wrong place; they act as if they're embarrassed that I am back, so they ignore me. Am I just imagining this, or is it true? Well, it doesn't make any difference, because I'm repeating the grade anyway. Another reason for me to repeat is the fact that this new class doesn't know what I have, and they act more natural.

Being with the von Moltkes so much recently has made me very happy. I get along with Dorothea very well, and by now our parents have become friends.

My dear, brave Maren, I pray that this time won't be too hard for you. Be strong, and think about the poem "Footsteps in the Sand," which you had once given me as a present. That helped me.

Until the next letter, I send you hugs.

Your Belli

P.S. Everyone here sends greetings!

MAY 25, 1982

Hello, dear Maren!

Just a minute ago I made a happy discovery; I found a ribbon I thought I had lost years ago. By my handwriting you can tell that my right arm is doing much better. Writing the letter yesterday was hard.

Now it is 11:00 a.m. and I am not in school, because of my arm. I could have gone if I had really wanted to, but I didn't. Just a month ago I wouldn't have dreamed of doing that.

This afternoon I will go downtown with Dorothea von Moltke. I look forward to that. When I sit around at home too much, I start to brood. Yesterday evening I constantly thought about my fourth chemotherapy session and, of course, I cried. I don't want to cry, but there is so little one can do against fear. My parents hurt so much when I cry. Then I always try to be happy again quickly, because otherwise my mom is so sad.

I rearranged my room. Now it's really cozy. I'm sitting on the couch, and in front of me I have my new little table with a candle, a teacup with accessories, a box of chocolates, and a slice of bread and butter, and I'm writing a letter to you.

Whenever you have time, please come and visit me. It would make me very happy.

Recently I have enjoyed writing letters. The "must" letters are still no fun, but I enjoy those letters in which I can really say something.

Did you take some good books with you? Just say the word, and I'll send you some. Do you know what I am reading now? Kalifornische Sinfonie *by Gwen Bristow. Didn't you read it together with Isi? It's supposed to be like* Gone with the Wind. *If so, I will certainly eat it up.*

Dear Maren, you will hear from me again soon. Keep your hopes up! We all think about you. Hugs.

Belli

69

he pain in your arm became worse. At one time it was so bad that the doctors suspected a fracture. The growth on your back had solidified to a knot the size of a golf ball. That must have put pressure on some nerves. The doctors at the Bonn Hospital examined you and contacted their colleagues in Cologne. They decided that your next series of treatments would have to begin sooner.

Your appointment had been for June 28 but that was too far away. We had to go back to Cologne on June 14.

The day before, Sascha was baptized. This date had been set a long time ago because you—by all means—were supposed to be there. And now you participated only with severe pain, but still you were able to be happy with your godchild. For us this was a difficult experience. We saw how much you were hurting, how you were clinching your teeth bravely so as not to dampen the mood of this lovely celebration.

Cologne, June 23, 1982

My dear Ines,

It looks as if Mom is writing this letter to you, because I'm dictating it to her. Unfortunately I had a setback that is terribly painful because now there's pressure on my nerves. For three days I've been having treatments, and that helps. It lessens the pain, but at the same time it puts me into a very unpleasant emotional state. What really helps me is the support of my parents and of a Canadian boy whom I met recently. It is incredible how considerate and understanding he is after we have known each other for only one week.

WE WILL MEET AGAIN IN HEAVEN

When I returned to the hospital in Cologne on June 14, they considered a radiation treatment. But I had to be helped as soon as possible because I couldn't stand the pain anymore, so they decided to go back to the old plan. Dr. Jaeger's visit gave me much courage. Right now I can no longer imagine how it would be to be free of pain and to feel well. Fortunately I am already being helped. Last night, for the first time in seven nights, I was able to sleep for five hours straight. Before that I had so much pain that I couldn't lie down or sit up during the nights even with four painkillers.

On June 13 we drove to Mannheim. We went to Siegfried's for the baptism of his youngest daughter. I became her godparent. The pins were also removed from my ankle joint. As you can see, we took full advantage of our last break between treatments.

My dear Ines, I send you a big hug and wish you all the best. Greetings to all your loved ones.

Isabell

After we arrived in Cologne this time several tests had to be done. The doctors and nurses in the main building, especially the ones in the X-ray section, already knew you well. Once again tissue was taken from the growth for a biopsy.

Nights were the worst. In spite of strong medication, you were unable to sleep because of the pain. This was your first setback. Until now we always thought only others would suffer setbacks. After all, we believed in miracles!

Again, it was human contact that motivated your fighting spirit most effectively. Jan would either visit you in Cologne or phone you. Thinking about him released enormous powers of resistance in you. He gave you the idea that you could "hang your pains in the cupboard," that the pain could be separated from your body, when you thought about something else. He was right: whenever you thought of him, you did not think about your pain.

Many younger patients were in the ward this time. You were best acquainted with Claudia, a young woman who wore beautiful scarves. She already had overcome several setbacks, and she gave you courage. She was a brave 25-year-old woman. Michael, a young student, was a new patient. He was perhaps lucky. The primary tumor had been discovered in the initial stage. He had a good chance of continuing his studies next semester. He was of great support to you. Together you played Stratego and listened to music.

Because this private ward of Dr. Jaeger's was located in a very old building with only one toilet and one shower, all of you had to cross the hallway, even during treatment and with your infusion rack. This was difficult, but it fostered contact among you. When they were feeling better, the patients would sit on chairs in the hallway. This was your communication center, where you could find out about everything that was going on in the ward.

On June 20 you were receiving chemotherapy again, and it really helped. Day by day your pain diminished. On one of those days you told Dr. L. how grateful you were that God let your body feel pain, because then you knew whenever the tumor was growing again. You had never heard or read about positive thinking before, but what a positive person you were!

On June 27 the treatments ended, and after three days you were allowed to come home. You had to remain in careful isolation, however, because of the low count of white cells in your blood. You also had a question: would you be allowed to kiss Jan if he came to visit? I didn't know, so I suggested that you ask Dr. L. He thought that it would be difficult to kiss with a mask over your mouth, and perhaps it would be better for you to make sure he didn't have a cold.

On July 3 we invited the entire Martin family to our home. After we ate, you young people went into your room while we talked to Hatty and Paul. We had a plan: according to Dr. Jaeger's estimate, we would be able to go on a vacation in August. We wanted to take Jan with us to a little vacation home in the Eifel area, a plateau in Western Germany. Before we could tell you, we had to talk it over with Hatty and Paul, and of course, with Jan too. On Sunday we asked Hatty and Paul. They were very much in favor of the plan.

On Monday evening Jan came to visit you. We asked him to come into our room first. (You were disappointed that he didn't come to see you first.) We told him about our plan, and we were careful to let him say no if he disagreed with it. He was very happy and went to tell you that he was going to come along.

All this took only twenty minutes, but your disappointment about Jan not seeing you first was too great. You became emotionally upset and were unable to recover. You had never been a moody girl, but this must have been one of the dreaded mood swings caused by the chemotherapy. Jan stood helpless in front of you and could not change your mood. I believe that on that evening he understood for the first time how sick you were, and he was deeply frightened.

As soon as he left, you wrote to him, again in English.

JULY 4, 1982

Dear Jan,

Now you are gone since half an hour, and I would like to thank you because you tried to help me so nice. You were a great help for me, and I promise you to try never to be like that again. I'll leave my illness in a bottle in the cupboard.

I must have been very strange because my whole family asked me what had happened.

You are a very close friend of mine because there are not many people besides my family I can speak so sincerely with. Sometimes I wonder why you like me. I have so many problems I have to live with, you can't do anything with me.

I have a very high opinion of your evening meetings with me because during that time there is always football and I believe you'd love to watch football.

It's nice to spend time with you. I was so sorry that you just had the two hours, I felt bad. Now, I feel much better again for the most part you were so kind to me.

I believe your whole family and you are very super people. We just know each other since two weeks and you already gave me so much power. It's nice to know such powerful people.

But I hope I won't only take. I will give you my help as

WE WILL MEET AGAIN IN HEAVEN

soon as I can and you'd like to take it. I hope Tuesday is
coming soon. I kiss you very soft and warm, enjoy that kiss!

Your Isabell

From then on Jan did not visit you as often, and your conversations were not as deep. When you asked him when he would come again, he was evasive. His answers became more vague, starting with "probably" or "perhaps." He began to withdraw from you. This was painful for you to accept. One time you told me: "Mom, I feel bad that Jan doesn't visit anymore, but I don't want to live with false illusions just in order to feel good."

During the break between treatments, we spent a very nice evening with Dr. L. and his wife, and Dr. Töbellius. We had invited them for a Japanese sukiyaki dinner. Töbi came a little early in order to talk to you. That evening Jan was already there. The young man was looked over very closely. The discussion was about sports—soccer especially (Jan was almost a professional)—and about American universities. Afterwards Dr. Töbellius (at that time we all called him Töbi) was a bit irritated and asked us: "Who is this self-confident, strong young man?" He was obviously concerned about Jan hurting you.

The evening was interesting and relaxed, the food was good, and the interest in Japan was genuine. Both Töbi and Dr. L. knew a lot about Japan. The conversation was open and intense.

After Jan left, you joined us. Töbi asked earlier why you wouldn't sit at our table. You looked just like your own self, wearing baggy trousers, slippers, with your shaved head uncovered. After Dr. L. and his wife left, we let the evening come to a harmonious end with Töbi and you.

On July 19 you had to go back to Cologne.

My Dear Doris,

I have received your very long letter and was so glad to read it.

Your trip must have been great. I'd love to do something like that myself. You really made me want to do it. Thank you very much for all the letters from America. That was really nice.

I have experienced a lot during my two-week break. I made contact with two of my teachers, Frau Niefindt and Frau Bell. Frau Bell visited me once. The chance to get in behind the scenes was especially interesting. And Frau Niefindt is a very interesting conversation partner as well, because she has undergone something similar to my condition and came through it well.

The last days at home were not easy for me. I had experienced a real trauma from my last chemotherapy, which I had to overcome by talking about it. Fortunately I had many people to help me. I did manage to develop a pretty good attitude, but sometimes I still become unstable.

Mrs. Martin, Jan's mother, has given me a bottle of water from Lourdes. She and her family are very religious, and they believe in this water because it is holy for Catholics. Once Mrs. Martin was very ill herself, and she is convinced that she was healed by that water. This present means a lot to me, because I know how much it means to Mrs. Martin. I make the sign of the cross twice a day with the water and somehow it builds me up.

What makes me happy sometimes is seeing how much I can enjoy little things. Today I sat in bed and dozed off and on. I believe that people on drugs have a similar feeling of euphoria.

I still need to tell you about the results of the examinations. The doctors could not yet make an official statement, but they found that the tumor has shrunk after having grown again. Dr. Jaeger said that he would continue to work for my complete recovery. I have never doubted that, and I never thought of anything else. At least that is very encouraging.

Dear Doris, enjoy the rest of your vacation time. Apparently I'll be home for the entire month.

The chemotherapy has started out well and is progressing better than the last time.

Greet everyone.

Your Belli

In July you had to go back for your seventh chemotherapy series. We were given the smallest and the darkest room of the ward, and there was not enough space for a second bed. At least there was a wing chair in the room. After Inge heard about that, she found a folding cot. Assi, a colleague of Dad's, brought it that same evening to Cologne. Setting up the cot every day wasn't much trouble, but the whole atmosphere was cramped, gloomy, and oppressive. The mood in the ward was very depressing as well.

A young woman from Greece, perhaps twenty years old, had just been admitted. She was unable to walk anymore, so we had no contact with her. The only person relating to her was a young Greek woman, a student who spoke German and who visited her daily. We tried to tell you as little as possible about that. But we could not prevent you from feeling that her condition was getting worse. An oxygen breathing apparatus was delivered to the ward and also a portable box, but we did not yet know what that was for. Two nights later we could hear the Greek student wailing and crying. The young woman had been relieved of her sufferings; she died far from home and her parents.

The next days on the ward were depressing. The door was sealed with tape from the outside. Everyone knew that the room was being disinfected. Your thoughts were full of gloomy questions. You wanted to know whether a dead body would be washed one more time. And by whom? When would it be placed in a coffin? In the ward or at the morgue? Talking with you required all our strength, and still we could not prevent you from falling into a deep depression. You did not want to live anymore.

Dr. Töbi spoke to us by telephone and found out about this. In the evening he drove to Cologne and immediately took over. He sent us parents out of the room by asking us whether he could talk to you in private. We knew nothing about the things he discussed with you, but when he called us back an hour and a half later, you were ready to continue the chemotherapy. How thankful we were to him!

The treatment worked, and your pains went away. In order to give you some diversion, I asked permission to take you in the car to a nearby park in the evening. Though it was summer we brought along a wool blanket and a pillow in case of wind. On the way we stopped at an Italian ice-cream parlor for two ice-cream cones. Then we were off to the Green Belt of Cologne.

Because I jogged almost daily I knew many beautiful spots. There was a bench right on the lake, not too far from the parking. The bench, lit by the evening sun, became *our* bench! We observed the swans and the ducks, every now and then a squirrel came by; we day-dreamed and waited until the evening sun had set. On our way back we stopped again at the Italian ice-cream parlor and picked up ice cream for every patient able to eat and for the nurses on night duty.

Many times we would gather the chairs in the hall-way and have a good talk. Not only did we bring refreshing ice cream, but a comforted heart as well. Instinctively you had the desire to pass that on to the other patients. Sometimes you had riddles for them to solve, or you told a funny story. You also had a few dry comments to make. We all enjoyed our ice cream, and we were thankful for your natural cheerfulness.

The next day your mood might be on the down-swing. On one such day that I will never forget—it was a humid, hot summer day—I managed to get you out of such a depression. I talked you into taking a stroll. (We gradually gained a few liberties at the ward in Cologne.) We had two hours off. When we left, you were very unhappy. Your fellow patients, those who were able to walk, were aware of that as they sat outside on the bench in the shade of the house.

We drove only three blocks to an area with nice boutiques. We walked into one of them, and we were lucky. The salesperson was friendly, and there were no other customers. You looked around and found a delightful dress, which you tried on right away. When the salesperson tried to help you, she discovered the taped hoses of your catheter, which peaked out at your collarbone. And the cotton scarf on your head slipped a little. It was a shock for her, but you handled the situation masterfully: "Don't worry, I'm only having chemotherapy!" you said. The salesperson quickly regained her composure.

You liked the dress, and you insisted that I buy something too. I did, but now I forgot what it was. You had fun and experienced new life. You asked, "Mom, do you think they'd recognize me if I came back to the ward wearing the new dress? They might all still be sitting outside on the bench!" Your eyes sparkling, we put the old clothes in a bag. You wore the new dress and tied your scarf elegantly. Back in the car you put on the sunglasses and some lipstick. We drove back very happy. The sparkling look in your eyes, the pride at having conquered the bad mood, and your cheerful smile reminded me of the old German proverb: "It doesn't take much to be happy, and whoever is happy is a king." All the others saw that in you and were happy for you.

This dress inspired you to think many pleasant thoughts. For which events would you wear it next? To whom would you show the dress? You managed to forget your pain for hours at a time, or, as Jan would have said, you put them in a bottle in the cupboard.

JULY 28, 1982

Dear Doris!

The chemotherapy ended yesterday, and right now I am receiving a blood transfusion because of my poor blood count. All in all, the news is incredibly good.

1. As you already know, all the examination results turned out to be very good.

2. As soon as my blood count improves, a new long-term treatment will be started, perhaps as soon as Friday. That means that I will get a shot only once a week, into the muscle in my bottom. This could last for three months if I take it well. Sometime in September there will be an intermediate exam that will determine the continuing treatment. This therapy will at least be much easier, allowing me to live quite normally.

3. I could even think about going back to school regularly. Many people have said that my new class is very nice, so I look forward to it.

Maybe my hair will grow back to the point where I don't have to wear a wig or a scarf. Just recently I discovered that wearing the scarf is much easier than this dumb wig.

Do you know that the Scholzes, the family of a classmate of mine, are very concerned about their father? Inge told me that he had a growth in his throat. The biopsy was positive, which means that he has cancer.

I wrote a letter to Isi about this, and I offered her advice on questions and problems that might arise. I also called her that evening. By then the results had shown that the cancer was at least treatable. I hope I helped her a bit by my call. I really had no choice because I had just written to tell her why I found the class's behavior so cowardly: they all just looked away from me! And I didn't want to act the same way toward her.

I hope that Herr Scholz is as lucky as I was in finding the right doctors.

We're racking our brains over our plans to visit you in August. If I attend school regularly, I could only visit during my break. Another possibility is seeing you the middle of September, when my class is on a field trip that I may not be allowed to take. Or you could come to see us if this is easier for you. I hope this works out.

During the past few days I didn't feel much like writing, but today it's fun.

Dear Doris, please say hello to your whole family from me. I hope I'll see you soon.

Belli

On July 30 we were allowed to go back home again with a great prospect: for the next three months you were to be treated as an outpatient. You would get an injection every two weeks, and in between you would have an outpatient exam. We were able to make plans for you to attend school and for a summer trip. The doctors had high hopes for Bleomycin, the injection you were to be given. You had heard that this treatment was often successful. On August 9, after the leukos were high enough, you got your first shot. Unfortunately, you didn't react to it well at all. You had attacks of fever and fits of shivering like never before. It was a good thing that Axel and Caroline came from Belgium and brought you some diversion.

Because of the school break, life was much quieter in Bonn. My friends helped out frequently. When you were feeling better, Löw took you to Oberwinter. Her two sons, Lippi and Patty, were there. You recuperated in the beautiful garden, you looked for new books in their large library, and you were grateful just to see something different. You also visited Josev and Jacqueline and Philippe and Johann. The two boys had a young visitor from Greece. These three charming, attractive young men sat in the garden with you. Jacqueline served exquisite refreshments, Johann played the guitar, and Philippe chatted with you about old times when you played tennis. You had tennis lessons with him back when you were ten. Sometimes Christian would come to see you, and together you played music tapes and dreamed of pleasant things.

You also received many letters. Dr. P., the pediatrician, wrote to you from the clinic in Cologne.

COLOGNE, AUGUST 11, 1982

My Dear Isabell,

Thank you very much for your dear letter. It's great that the treatments proceeded without complications. I'm glad that you have the prospect of fourteen weeks of outpatient treatment. I hope that you respond well to Bleomycin and that you won't experience any side effects.

It's an excellent idea to take a vacation now, not only for your parents, but for you too. I know all too well how much a stay in the clinic, the treatments, and especially all the waiting can get to us and how tiring they are. Then it is especially important to take full advantage of the times of rest to experience beautiful things, joy, and new impressions. The more we can take in, the less we will be troubled by unconscious, as well as conscious, worries. For that reason I wish you a beautiful vacation.

If you want to go back to school, take it easy, especially at the beginning. Don't be too ambitious or disappointed. Some things will be different from before. Your sickness has not only challenged your body, but your mind, your thoughts, emotions, and feelings as well—and that is quite different from the challenge of school. You have had other problems and ways of thinking. Switching back to school will at first be a bit difficult, and also adjusting to the class as a group of people. They have had a different development from yours. You will need to be patient and calm with your-self and with the others before the two worlds come together again. This psychological process is quite normal, and it shouldn't scare you. I wish you strength and patience for this too.

But first of all, I hope you have a happy vacation. I think about you, and I wish you well from the bottom of my heart.

Ulrike P.

AUGUST 15, 1982

Dear Doris,

By now your school year has started again. Your visit with me was great.

Since then quite a few things have happened. I received my first Bleomycin injection; unfortunately I did not take it well at all. I had a temperature of 104 degrees, and then I had severe chills. All of this subsided quickly however, and I hope that I'll respond better to the next shots.

All in all, this is still a thousand times better than being in the hospital. I also have many visitors.

Dear Doris, I'm sorry, but I don't feel like writing a letter. I just wanted to say hello.

Please don't be angry at me for writing so little.

Goodbye.

Belli

On August 16 we were allowed to go to Oberlahnstein for five days. We stayed at a good hotel with vacation facilities. Never before had we as a family with three children stayed in such an expensive hotel. But we wanted it to be the finest possible under these circumstances. We were not allowed to drive very far, and a hospital had to be close by for monitoring your blood count.

For you the most beautiful thing was that we parents could have a little vacation. You watched with joy when we played tennis with the boys. In spite of the pain in your arm, you were permitted to swim. You were happy like a fish in the water. After all, you were a good swimmer, and two legs and one arm were enough for swimming. You also played table tennis with Christian and Matthias. They put you on a chair and hit the balls within your reach, because walking was hard for you. That was cheating a little, but you and the boys had fun. We also took a beautiful steamboat ride up the Lahn River and down the Rhine. The other passengers did not notice that you frequently had to take your temperature. A bout of fever would mean that you couldn't sit in the open but had to go inside. Everything went well. The boys, too, were very happy.

On the day before we left, we invited the Martin family and Jan. It wasn't easy to convince Dad of this plan. Jan was going back to college in Canada at the beginning of September. We didn't know if you would ever meet again, and we didn't want a sad ending. You wanted very much to see Jan. Hatty understood this right away. It was a harmonious day and a relaxed good-bye with the possibility of meeting again at Christmas when Jan would visit Germany.

On August 23 we had to go back for the next injection. Extensive examinations were scheduled, a computerized tomography and an X-ray of the lungs. The director of radiology examined you personally. He was a tall, stately man with white hair. He did not look like someone who would be upset easily. After the examination he came to me and all he said was: "The therapy has to be stopped immediately. I will talk to Dr. L.!"

You had just received your second injection and Dr. Jaeger was on vacation! The director of radiology was pale; for him too you had become more than just a patient. I had to fight back my tears. I don't know why, but in his concerned look I saw that he had discovered something terrible in your lungs. At that moment all hope for a medical miracle was gone.

The doctors discussed your case. You needed a different treatment as soon as possible. A bed had to be made available, and Dr. Jaeger had to be informed. The results of the second biopsy finally came in as well. Two institutions had analyzed it independently, and their results were not identical. They agreed in diagnosing the primary tumor as a ganglionic neoplasm, a malignant tumor.

This time we counted the days until we could return to Cologne. We finally had a bed on August 30.

AUGUST 30, 1982

Dear Doris,

This is only a short and scrawly letter, because I'm having a lot of pain again. Unfortunately I had another setback. The outpatient therapy has not worked out.

For the next five days I'll be having a very tough treatment so that the tumor will get smaller again. I'm glad that something is being done now, because this constant pain is terrible.

You won't hear from me before Sunday because the treatments will last that long.

Dear Doris, I hope you had a good start at school. I didn't have a chance to start at all.

Say hello to your mother.

Belli

his treatment was especially severe but you fought hard. You had intended to go back to school the beginning of September—to your new class. But we had to give up that idea. However, your new class did not forget you. They got in touch with you. Frau Keller, your new teacher, and your new classmates, all struggled along with you. At first they sent letters, then Frau Keller came in person to Cologne, and a while later some students ventured out to visit you as well. This was very encouraging to you.

SEPTEMBER 2, 1982

Dear Isabell,

I hope you have received all the greetings your new class sent. I would like to—we would all like to—give you more than just a few written words. We'll do that later when you return home. I hope you feel how often and how much I keep thinking about you. Until now I knew you only from your morning greeting in the schoolyard whenever I was on duty: "Good morning, Frau Keller!" It was good to talk with you more in depth when I visited you last week. This conversation gave me much to think about.

Carry on with all your courage! Sometimes we can relieve the psychological burden of a person a little by just being there and by being ourselves. You will have to endure the physical pain on your own when medical treatment cannot alleviate it. But I firmly believe that you can gain strength and confidence by knowing that many people in their thoughts are with you in your hospital room and are trying to imagine what you are suffering.

*My thoughts reach out to you. Now I hesitate, because
what I feel appears so shallow when expressed in words. Let
me therefore tell you what you already know: we are all with
you and we hope that the Spirit, with all of its powers, will
triumph over our physical helplessness.*
*I will visit you as soon as it is possible. Your parents will
let me know.*
Heartfelt greetings.

Ruth Keller

Björn came to visit you at this time. He had been
an admirer of yours, and he was waiting for a
response from you. But as nice as he was, he was
not your type. On the day he came, you weren't feeling
well. Björn nevertheless sat at your bed for three hours
and took touching photos of you. No other pictures captured the atmosphere of the ward in Cologne so well.

Another source of strength was offered by Bud, a psy-
chologist at the American school. He was your former
partner in tennis tournaments at the club, and he wanted
to help you. He talked to me and suggested that relaxation and hypnosis exercises might strengthen your
immune system. We were suspicious about hypnosis, but
we had much confidence in Bud. I asked Dr. L. whether
hypnosis might alter your personality. "Hypnosis would
alter her teeth before it would change Isabell's charac-
ter!" was his answer. We also asked Dr. Jaeger, who told
me that anything can help if you believe in it. I just had
to promise him that all his medical instructions would

be strictly followed. For us that was self-evident. At this point we even tried all kinds of scientifically tested nutrition products. In such situations one tries to take advantage of every opportunity that comes along. Bud was allowed to go ahead.

He insisted on being alone with you in the room. I had to make sure nobody would come in and disturb you. Again, I sat on a chair outside, at the door, like a watchdog. One hour later Bud came out the door. He had activated your healthy cells so that they would fight the cancer cells. After Bud left, you gave me a charming account: "You know, Mom, at first it was quite pleasant. I was supposed to dream about things I love to do the most. Then he spoke to my cancer cells as if he wanted to demolish them. At the end he mentally took me swimming and to the tennis court. I did him that favor!" You took all this with good humor. Bud did help you, however. From then on you talked almost daily to your "evil cancer cells," fighting against them. Bud had activated your fighting spirit.

SEPTEMBER 10, 1982

Dear Doris,

The chemotherapy is over. It was really hard, but worked wonderfully. My pain is bearable, and I can go home tomorrow for two or three weeks. I didn't expect that at all. After this break the same series will be repeated.

So, now you have a general summary of what happened. Mentally I am doing great right now. I am incredibly lucky, cheerful, and eager to venture out.

*Björn visited me last Monday. That was quite some-
thing. He stayed for three hours, and I was happy that he
came to see me.*

*Naturally it ended the way it had to. He asked me
whether I loved him. I gently told him no. I hope he got over
it. Besides that, Monday evening was really fun because
there were so many young patients in the ward.*

*Dear Doris, greet your mother for me. I hope we will be
together soon.*

Belli

O

n September 11 we drove back home.

Some new classmates came to visit you one after the
other. That made you very happy. One time—when I got
home—you had three or four girls from your new class
visiting you. Scented candles were lit in your room.
Somebody must have brought them. I believe Ingund
brought a guitar. You were all sitting on the floor and
singing, even though you were critically ill. I worried
about your lungs, but at the same time I was very happy
that it was possible for you to live a little.

I took you several times to Mrs. Gipson, a friend of
Hatty's. There you could watch films on video. She got
you every film you wanted to see. I remember two films
that fascinated you in particular. One was *On Golden
Pond,* starring Katherine Hepburn and Henry Fonda. The
film shows the everyday life of an older married couple
who were fighting a lively running battle. When you

came home, you said: "Mom, this film shows the two of you in about thirty years!" The other film, *Caesar and Cleopatra* starring Elizabeth Taylor, moved you very much. I watched the last half hour together with you. Cleopatra, a great woman, wanted to die with dignity and not as a slave. For her the fatal snakebite was the only means of achieving that.

You thought more and more about death. Dr. Töbi came over one evening. We all sat in the living room. Dad was there too. I could sense that you had some burning questions that you could discuss only with Töbi. I left the room and hoped Dad would do the same. But that didn't even cross his mind. After five minutes I drew Dad out of the room by saying that he had a phone call. Then I asked him to leave the two of you alone. He thought that was extremely impolite, but he stayed with me.

You took full advantage of that half hour alone with Töbi. You wanted to know how death from your kind of illness would take place. (You always faced people and the future head-on.) Töbi took away your fear of pain, and that gave you hope of dying in dignity.

SEPTEMBER *17, 1982*

Dear Doris,

I just looked at the correspondence of the last four weeks. Your pack of letters was so thick that it made me very happy to have such a good friend. The tapes were a super idea, especially the comedians. Both are very good.

As Dad may have told you already on the phone, I am not doing so well at the moment. I am very much afraid that the treatments may not work. If that happens, I won't want to be treated anymore, because there is no benefit, only the pain of the treatments. At the moment I am very discouraged and depressed, because the severe pain came back almost immediately. This therapy was especially difficult, and still I have pain.

I am also afraid about how I will die. It's so cruel. Sometimes I can't breathe, and sometimes I can't move. And I want so much to live!

Dear Doris, give your mom my love.

Belli

SEPTEMBER 21. 1982

Dear Belli,

Thank you very much for your letter. It was very, very open. I'll try to answer you just as openly. That leaves me a bit perplexed. I could just write about the weather or about other things, but then I wouldn't be responding to what you have written, and I don't want to ignore your concerns. I would like to help you somehow.

Only one thing comes to mind that I think will really help you. It's hard for me to express it in a way that will not appear as useless theory. Perhaps you think it is easy for me to talk because I'm not in your situation. But I'll try to tell you and hope it will really help.

As you know, I believe in Jesus Christ. I believe that he can help everyone in every situation. Unfortunately, there's a question for which I have no answer. I don't know why he allows you to suffer such pain. That is simply a mystery. Therefore, it may be hard to believe that God loves everyone. That seems impossible, but I am firmly convinced of it—perhaps just because Jesus had to suffer so much pain on the cross. That is why he can understand you better than anyone else. He can help because he knows and understands you so well, even if we can't know why he allows so much evil to happen.

You may think that I can talk easily about God's love because I don't know any real pain. You're right, but there are many other people who believe in God in spite of their sufferings. I think for instance about Joni Earakson. That's why I want to go on writing to you, even if I have not suffered nearly as much as you have.

I like one Bible verse very much. Jesus says: "I have come that they might have life and have it more abundantly." At first this sentence looks ridiculous or even wrong. Pain like yours does not seem to be part of "abundant life." However, God has very different standards, which are hard for us to understand. When God talks about life, he does not mean life that we find desirable, for instance luxury, entertainment, or other things. God offers us a different life: life with fulfillment, with meaning, with inner peace and joy. He offers this kind of life to every one of us. It's up to us whether we trust in him and accept his offer. A passage of the letter to the Romans (Romans 8:34-38) says that nothing, not death or life or any other power can ever separate us from the love of God. This means that nothing can destroy a life given by God. Life with God will never end. It will last forever, because it is not determined from the outside. This means that you can live, regardless of whether or not the therapy is successful. God is always with you. He gives you strength, strength to overcome your fear.

*Dear Belli, this is what I wanted to tell you. I hope it
was not too condescending and theoretical. I will remember
you in my prayers. I wish you the very best, God's blessings,
and with all my heart I hope treatments are successful.*

Doris

P.S. My mother sends her warmest greetings.

O n September 19, 1982, just two weeks after you finished
your last treatment, you had to return to Cologne. You
had so much pain in your knee that you were able to walk
only with crutches.

95

SEPTEMBER 19, 1982

Dear Doris,

*I am back in the hospital, and I am not doing very well.
The chemotherapy has been changed, and now I have to
throw up quite often.*

But I wanted to thank you for your letter.

*The Protestant pastor just came in. He supposedly
wanted to see me since November of 1981 but never came.*

*During these treatments Dad has been with me. Right
now he is a patient himself, because he wants to have a
complete physical.*

*Dear Doris, don't be angry that I am writing so little.
Greet everyone for me.*

Belli

Dear Doris,

I received both of your letters and the tree bark as well. That was a pretty clever idea to send a piece of bark by mail; the post office had no choice but to deliver it.

I will soon have a subclavian catheter inserted. Until then I want to write as many letters as I can.

The last chemotherapy has brought almost no relief at all. That is why some new treatments are being tried. I hope very much that I will respond to it. If those treatments don't work, I will really be scared. The pain, especially in my lungs, will be even worse.

Dear Doris, I don't know how I will do in those treatments that will last for ten days, so I can't tell you how soon you will hear from me again.

Until then, all the best. I don't think I will make it to Oberursel for a while. Goodbye.

Belli

P.S. Greet your mother.

The Platinex therapy was new. We were informed about the risks of permanent damage caused by this kind of therapy. It could result in deafness and destruction of the kidneys if your body was not constantly flushed with liquids. Every day we had to collect the urine of the previous 24 hours, and get you to drink three or four quarts of liquid. But you did not want to drink anything because you felt so nauseous. We had to keep a record of every cup of liquid you drank and of every drop of urine you passed. Even for a healthy, tough person that would have been extremely annoying. How much harder it was for a patient plagued with pain, who had to manage every walk to the toilet using crutches and dealing with an infusion rack. You could not do that by yourself anymore. At least two persons had to be with you. But you wanted to keep your mobility as long as possible.

This therapy demanded of you and of us the utmost in willpower and discipline. Almost always you felt nauseous, and you couldn't look at food, much less smell it. Even for brushing my teeth, I had to use the patients' bathroom. Dad and I had to have our breakfast and coffee in the hallway. When Dad came after work on Friday to relieve me, I was almost at the end of my rope. But how much worse you must have felt. When Dad said goodbye to me, he said: "Try to get some rest!"

I sat down in the car and began to cry uncontrollably. As I drove to the highway, I felt like driving far away, anywhere, to a place where I could forget everything. As I saw the signs along the highway, I thought about my friend, Lou, in Antwerp and my brother, Siegfried, in Mannheim. Yes, I had to see one of them; with either one I could feel safe. But what about Matthias and Christian? They were waiting for me at home, and they needed me too. They didn't try to escape. So was it fair for me to run away? I went home to the boys and talked with them. Both were very supportive and advised me to leave for the weekend. I called Siegfried and Ulli that evening, and Saturday morning I drove to Mannheim.

That was a refreshing weekend. I felt comforted by love and understanding. Playing tennis and bicycle riding were stimulating and diverting. Saturday evening we went out to dine in style. In our talks we were close to you and Dad, but we also discussed other things. It felt so good—this care for both body and spirit! When I returned home Sunday evening, I could bring some of this care back for the boys. When I changed shifts with Dad very early Monday morning, I could offer you new courage and new things to talk about.

One ray of hope in these days was Jacob, whom we called "Sunnyboy." He was a young, attractive, charming medical student. For this series of treatments he was on night duty, and that turned out to be a lot of fun. Every evening Jacob came dashing to work in his sports car, probably earned by his hard work. What amazed us was his big heart for everything human, in addition to his good looks and his charm. Every evening he came into your room and tried to cheer you up. I couldn't go to the bathroom often and long enough in order to let the two of you be together. In the evenings I had even fewer opportunities to leave the room.

Sunnyboy did not hide his affection for you at all, though he always maintained his professional stance. Every day you looked forward to his being on duty. You also showed him the latest photos Siegfried had taken. He asked for one of them. That made you very happy. Doris also came from Oberursel to visit you.

Dear Doris,

What a surprise to see you standing by my bed when I woke up.

One day later I received your tape. Thank you very, very much. It has already given me four beautiful, pleasant hours.

Yesterday my therapy was stopped because my leukocyte count had dropped drastically, but that was all right with me.

Do you know which of my teachers wrote to me? Frau Hertwek! Remember her? In fifth and sixth grades we had her for biology.

I am so glad when people from everywhere write letters, call, and visit me. Today Frau Keller visited me for the second time. So far, five classmates have visited me. I'm surprised by so much warmth.

Dear Doris, I hope you can come to visit me during your fall vacation.

Greet your mother. Goodbye.

Belli

You had a growing need to put your thoughts down on paper. You wrote letters whenever your physical condition allowed it. One day your new classmates brought you a little notebook bound in Chinese silk. On the cover it said *Diary*, and it contained only blank pages. Your first question was: "What should I do with this?" I answered: "You could write down your thoughts." In Cologne you started.

On October 1 the Platinex therapy was discontinued early, because the count of your leukos was too low. You had less pain, however, and the X-rays showed improvements. We were relieved.

One evening Dad and I were invited over by some friends. This gave us an opportunity to think about something else. At around nine o'clock p.m. you called us because you had earaches. Dad immediately drove to Cologne and stayed.

The following Sunday an alarming piece of news made its rounds on the floor: your friend Claudia's blood-profile was deteriorating. After surviving chemotherapy, she had overcome leukopenia. Yesterday she still sat with us in the hallway. Today Claudia's brothers were called and asked to come from a distance. At first we tried to conceal these developments from you, but that was impossible. On Monday you met one of Claudia's brothers in the hallway and asked him why she didn't come out of her room. Michael, the young student, was also back for treatment at the ward, and he finally tried to tell you gently about Claudia. It was shocking for all of us but especially for you. Of all the patients on the ward you felt closest to Claudia.

Sister Elisabeth, the nurse, tried to get you released from the ward, so you wouldn't have to witness Claudia's death. She died on Tuesday night. She found peace, but you tell the rest of the story much better.

OCTOBER 15, 1982

My very dear Dr. P.,

I have been released from the hospital for four days, and already I have so much to tell you. Actually I could have written to you every single day, each time with a new problem or a new emotional state. Everything happened so fast, one thing after another. It took me this long to digest and accept everything.

One thing at a time.

On Tuesday I was released, and both Mom and I were emotionally weighed down because Claudia, a young woman on the ward, was dying. By now Claudia has passed away. For my parents and me this was very sad. We liked Claudia very much. She had given me so much courage during a critical time in June. She was twenty-seven years old and had cancer in her lymph glands. She had been treated for three years but without significant success. At times she felt quite well, and I believe that she had a tremendous will to live and that she was incredibly courageous. But the cancer won.

Sister Elisabeth, a nurse on the ward, tried to keep all this away from me because she was afraid that my condition, which had just stabilized, would suffer another downturn. On Monday morning Claudia's brother told me everything, and I am grateful for that. I don't know how I would have taken the news of Claudia's death if I had been informed just one day later. Claudia died Tuesday night, and thanks to Sister Elisabeth, who tried everything conceivable, I was released just before Claudia's death. I would have found out about it sooner or later, but Sister Elisabeth spared me from witnessing it. Her mother, both of her brothers, and a

101

friend bravely accepted Claudia's destiny, and I admire them for that. Everyone on the ward fell into a depression as a result.

I could not understand why Claudia's condition deteriorated so quickly. She had unexpectedly relapsed into another leukopenia just after recovering from a series of treatments. So she couldn't have any more treatments. Just seven days before she died, she was running around and sitting on the bench with her brother, and all of a sudden she wouldn't get out of bed anymore. Soon after this she died.

How can this happen so fast? For her death was the worst thing—but in another way, the best. Still, I can't understand it. Even as I left on Tuesday, this upset me very much. I talked with my parents all about death, about why I am afraid to die, and if I will die soon like Claudia. After about an hour my father told me that I wore them out by thinking about death all the time. I realized that this was inconsiderate and self-centered of me. My parents didn't like it at all. It must have been a protective measure for me to talk about death so often, but as a result I trampled on their nerves and on their love.

At that moment I wanted to give up and not fight anymore, but fortunately nobody asked me. I thought that I would die soon, and I was quite depressed, like in my worst times. I tried to get myself together again after my father asked me to. I managed to do that pretty well. During the night I had to throw up once. Before that my lungs hurt badly, but afterwards I was all right.

On Wednesday morning I cleaned my room a little, and I muddled along until three in the afternoon, when I had visitors. In the course of the day my pain increased. In the evening the pain became so bad that I was very upset again, but we didn't do much about it. My entire right side was

*hurting all the time. On Thursday we had an appointment
with Dr. Töbellius, although we would have seen him anyway. My pain got so severe that I could hardly walk. This
was incredibly disappointing, because the pain was back
right away and it was so bad. I became quite hopeless
because I couldn't imagine why the pain returned so soon.
After all, the X-rays looked so good. Dr. Töbellius advised
us to start new treatments immediately.*

*I couldn't figure out the whole situation and why I
needed to go back to Cologne. I was in such a bad mood.
Claudia's fight lasted for three years and she lost. And for
me this was the shortest break ever between treatments.*

*On the other hand, I had this awful pain that could be
alleviated only by treatments. I was crushed. Again I had
planned too far ahead. I was so, so—I can't find a word for
it. I just didn't want to believe that I would have to get back
on that treadmill. I was so worn out!*

*There have been some new developments, however. I can
begin the next therapy session very soon in the Bonn hospital. Suddenly I'm happy. I was ready to go there voluntarily.
I have pain again, but now I don't feel so hopeless anymore.
Cologne would have been hard to take this time.*

*Mom thinks that the pain could have a psychological
basis: as soon as I was back home—boom—I had pain.*

*Perhaps it would be good if you could talk to our
family—individually or however it may work out. Mom and
I would like that, and it would be very good for my brothers.
I don't believe that they still really understand my illness.*

*I have to talk to my father about that. Dear, dear Dr. P.,
I can only admire how you carry all your burdens!*

I wish you all the best.

Isabell

Dear Isabell,

Today was very strenuous. You'll notice that in my handwriting, but I do want to write to you today.

Your long and open letter made me very happy. I was able to imagine quite well how you must have felt. Thank you so much for confiding in me.

You know, Isabell, I think about you every day. I'm sending you a big bouquet of best wishes. These thoughts about you get even more intense, when I imagine how you are feeling. I am so glad that you regained your courage after the distressing experience with Claudia. Out of my own experience I know how difficult this can be. I believe one should indeed talk about one's own fears openly and often. Don't be too hard on yourself. That consumes too much of your energy, which could be put to better use in fighting the tumor.

If you, my dear Isabell, or any of your loved ones would like to talk to me, I'm ready at any time. Just let me know.

You have been in the hospital for two days now. Along with you, I hope that the problem in your knee joint is diagnosed soon and that it can be treated effectively. But don't lose your patience, as difficult as that may be. Often only time will show what actually happened to a part of the body.

Bruzky, my cat, wants to help write this letter. He repeatedly gnaws at my pen, studies my handwriting, and hisses when I pull the paper away. I will send you a photo of him so that you can see the little monster for yourself. He sends you warm greetings.

I also greet you with all my heart. Let me hear from you again soon. My best wishes are with you. You certainly don't need to admire me, because you are just as brave.

Ulrike P.

iegfried visited us again with Ulli and Sascha. They wanted to bring us some joy and relaxation—and no stress or work. They brought their favorite foods with them, all prepared. During the whole weekend I was not allowed to go into the kitchen. Siegfried took some beautiful photos of you. He also made a close-up of your lips. Sweet little Sascha and her natural love gave you much comfort.

During these days we put up a folding bed in our living room. We wanted you to have the nicest room with the best view of the garden, and we wanted you to be at the center of the family. During the nights I slept next to you in the living room.

When Sascha had her first birthday, you wanted to do something nice for her.

105

OCTOBER 17, 1982

My dear little Sascha,

Even though you are still too little for this letter, I hope that some day it will be meaningful for you.

I really value physical and mental health right now, and I hope with all my heart that you will have good health.

You are just one year old, and I hope you will have many happy years ahead of you. My wish is that you will have as little trouble in your life as possible.

Unfortunately I have been able to see very little of you during your short life. But your charm and your happiness have captured me anyway.

I hope that you like the ball we are giving to you. When we were little, we also had such a ball and we loved to play with it.

I wish you a beautiful and interesting first birthday and all the love in the world.

Three cheers to you from all of us!

Isabell

*O*n October 16, 1982, Jan called from Canada and talked with you for a long time. He wanted to return to Germany for Christmas to visit his parents and to see you as well. He tried to renew your strength.

Sunday evening Dr. Töbi came over once more. He brought something for you: a little old steel block with a coat of arms engraved on it and an inscription: "Greetings from the Egerland." We did not know the origins of this steel block. He gave you this gift "out of the blue," as he put it. Since then I have had it polished, and I gave it back to Töbi as a keepsake.

On Monday, October 18, we went to the hospital in Bonn. You were anxious before the treatments. One of us always stayed with you at night. The doctors tried to alleviate the pain in your knee by radiation treatment, but that did not help. On October 22 the second Platinex treatment began. You were allowed to take one more bath before the catheter was inserted. We were by ourselves in the large bathroom on the ward. There you asked if I thought that you were dying. I told you that I was still hoping for a miracle, but you sensed that my faith had diminished.

Fortunately we had many friends who helped us talk with you. Inge offered you books about death, but that didn't work very well. You didn't want anything that heavy. The three teachers—Frau Keller, Frau Bell, and Frau Niefindt—were confronted with quite a few of your anxious questions, and together with you they tried to search for honest answers. You still wanted to make Christmas presents. You wanted to embroider and knit blankets, in spite of the pain in your arm. Brigitte and Hatty planned with you, brought everything you needed, and helped you.

Dr. Töbellius once saw me in the hallway and asked if he could talk with me. He told me that four days after you completed your treatments, he was leaving for his vacation. He would be gone for four weeks. He had planned a long trip that could not be postponed. He also told me that he had never been so close to a young patient and that it would be hard for him to leave.

You accepted it without complaint. You even wished him a much-needed vacation. The following day Sister Ulrike brought you two photographs of him. With Dr. Petri and Dr. Kern you were in the best of hands, but for you nobody could replace Töbi.

On October 31 the treatments ended, but the pain remained. You were given a device by which you could adjust the dosage of the painkiller Dipidolor yourself. That helped. Now the pain became partly bearable, but it took some skill to adjust the right dose of medication.

One night there was a scary incident. Dad was with you, and he phoned me at about eleven p.m. "I think Belli is dying. Please come immediately!"

"Have you called the doctor?" I asked.

"Sister Ulrike has notified the doctor on night duty."

I had neither the phone number nor the address of Dr. Petri, but I did have the number of the second head physician. She lived close by and came to the hospital immediately. Never before had I driven to the hospital so fast. On the ward I met Sister Ulrike, who told me that you were still alive and that your condition had stabilized. Apparently you had set the dosage of Dipidolor too high, and as a result your circulatory system collapsed.

You had delusions and thought that you were going to heaven. But that was not the way you wanted to die. You had accepted the fact that you were going to die, but not like that. That was not going to be your farewell.

Dr. Töbellius came in the next morning and calmed you down. He visited you often now because he planned to leave in two days. He avoided everything that may have suggested a final farewell. Whenever he came to talk however, he could not find a chance to be alone with you. Somebody was always there. You had to assure him several times that you were going to behave, at least until he came back in four weeks. On November 5 he left for Tibet.

Dad often told you stories in these days to comfort you. When he would leave, he would write a "little story for Belli" on a plastic slate, like this one.

"Why," asked the little girl, "do *I* always have to help mother?"

The mother answered: "Because you are a girl, and girls like to help better than boys!"

"But I like to help exactly as much as boys do, and the boys don't help at all!" Confused, the little girl went to her father: "Dad, I help just as the boys and you do, and Mom does everything. Am I nice?"

Or another story.

> Dad is discontented because Mom is not there. The little girl is worried. "Dad, come on, we'll have a really good time now. You set the table, and I will help you. Then you can quickly go to the store, and I will dry the dishes. When Mom gets back home, she'll be happy." Dad is irritated and goes on the balcony to smoke a cigarette. The little girl nags. Dad realizes that she is right. The table is set.
>
> Mom comes home, everyone is happy, and they all accuse Dad of being a "stinker." "Smoking is unhealthy!" they say. Once again Dad promises to improve.

Dad had to give a lecture in Berlin on November 5. I encouraged him to take Matthias with him and to stay over the weekend at the home of his sister, your Aunt Friedel, and her husband. Matthias had a birthday on November 8, and that would give him and Dad an opportunity to do something special together. They were uneasy when they left, but everything went well.

On this weekend you had many visitors. Friday, the hospital pastor from Bonn came unannounced. Grandma and I were with you. He said that he really had no time, but he wanted to see you anyway. You asked: "Why?" He said that he had asked at the ward who the sickest patient was. You replied: "You mean who would be next in line to die? You may be at the right place, but this is not the right time." He never came to visit you again.

Saturday, Siegfried and Ulli arrived once more with Sascha. That made you very happy. Jacob, the medical student, wanted to visit you again Sunday afternoon. You were very excited, but your only fear was that Dad and Matthias would be back from Berlin too soon. Jacob came from Aachen just to visit you. When he arrived, I quickly drove home and when I returned, he was still there. Fortunately, Dad and Matthias arrived later. They told us about how hard Aunt Friedel and her husband tried to cheer them up, but their efforts were not successful. In their thoughts, Dad and Matthias were always with you.

Dr. Kern was on night duty. In the evening he stopped by again for his "Gummi-bear visit." You always had something to offer your visitors. He loved Gummi-bears. If he had a little time, he would sit with you and devour one or two of them. You asked him what it was like to be on night duty, and if he could get any sleep. He said that you could wake him tomorrow at twenty minutes to eight.

From then on your first thought in the morning was: "I have to wake up Dr. Kern!" The two of you developed a cordial relationship. Dr. Burbi came to visit you quite often as well. He was working on another ward, but he got along well with Dr. Kern. They even visited you together. You had named your little hedgehog "Burbi." Maren made him for you out of a piece of fur that she had given you last Christmas. You decided that Dr. Burbi should have this hedgehog to remember you.

On November 8 Matthias had his birthday. You were already very sick. Grandma baked a cake and waited at home. For two hours we were allowed to take you home in a wheelchair and with crutches. Your arrival was Matthias' biggest joy. He and Dad carried you up the stairs. You sat at the table covered in blankets. This must have been hard for Matthias to see, yet we were all happy that you could be there.

In the evening we returned to the hospital. You didn't want to stay at home overnight because you needed the immediate protection of the doctors and the feeling that they would be instantly available. It was sweet of you to send me back home that evening. You wanted me to sleep at home. Dad had to leave in the afternoon for a lecture, and you did not want Matthias to be alone on his birthday. After I settled you in for the night, I left you with a tender kiss.

The next morning you were anxiously waiting for me because you were feeling bad. You had pain everywhere, and soon you developed a fever. Was the fever caused by the tumor, or was there something else? Actually, you had a bacterial pneumonia. But you did not give up. You did not want to die of pneumonia. After all, you had promised Dr. Töbellius that you would behave. You had fought the tumor so far, and should you now be defeated by pneumonia? You overcame this as well!

At that time Dr. Kern had asked me when we were alone how I managed to stand all this. I confessed to him that for more than twenty years—since my mother's death—I had a phobia about cancer. Every day something else would hurt me, and I didn't trust myself to talk about it to anyone, not even my father. In my fears I imagined all kinds of situations. However, in my fears it was always I who had cancer! For a year now, since fate struck you, I lost this fear. After that conversation I was quite upset. Dr. Kern gave me something to calm me down, and then I went back to your room. You needed me now. I could cry later.

November 11, 1982, was a special day. One year before, you had been admitted to the Bonn hospital. Three years before, Grandpa had died on St. Martin's Day. Something special was in order for today. We decided to have a surprise for the nurses on the ward. After all, this was St. Martin's Day, and we had lived with you for a whole additional year. A year ago we counted the days. At a bakery I ordered a Martin Man be baked three feet tall. The old baker Schulz on the corner made the Martin Man himself out of gingerbread dough. He decorated it so nicely with almonds that the nurses hesitated to eat it.

Brigitte was with you in the afternoon. We didn't know that Valerie and the children from the neighborhood planned to visit you and sing for St. Martin's Day. You were overwhelmed by this kindness. Brigitte called me right away. Over the phone I could hear the St. Martin songs, as well as your sobbing. You remembered when you yourself had made the rounds to sing for St. Martin's Day. Still this was a great joy for you.

Sibylle Pagenkopf, your former tennis coach, came to visit you again. You remembered the highlights of your tennis career, to which you said goodbye in thought.

Lou came one more time with her whole family from Belgium. By now we had to schedule visiting hours, because your time and your energies were limited. When they said goodbye to you, everyone tried to schedule another visit. No one wanted to give the impression that this would be the last goodbye.

Marie came from Belgium twice in these days (she had gone home for the summer). Each time her visit was a festival. The first time you gave her a scarf and a hat you had knitted as a present. Her happiness gave you so much joy in return. On the evening of her first visit—it was in October—I went to the tennis banquet with Marie. Both of us had played in the summer tournament, and you insisted that we go. You wanted us to pick up our trophy. Two weeks earlier you had considered attending the tennis banquet yourself and wondered what dress you should wear. In the same conversation, you asked what a person would wear in a casket. In a single hour you wondered about a party dress and burial clothes. At that time we refused to participate in your thoughts. That's all we could do.

Marie's second visit was unforgettable. It was Sunday. Dad, I, the boys, and Marie were with you. You were happy and got along with Marie so well. You told her about Jacob and about your newly discovered joy in flirting. Both of you made plans. If you didn't die, you would both make a trip on a luxury liner and you would have a great time. "And then, Marie, we'll flirt with all the men, won't we?" you said. We all had to laugh.

Someone knocked on the door. Dr. Petri and Dr. Kern came in. Both of them were off duty but wanted to visit you anyway. They were a bit startled because we were laughing so hard. "Doctors, please come in!" you said. "You are in the room of a very sick patient, but we're having fun anyway. May I offer you a cookie?" The two doctors quickly recovered from their surprise and chatted cheerfully with us.

Meanwhile you had figured out how to regulate the Dipidolor safely so the level of your pain was bearable. The only treatment at the time was the radiation of your knee.

You talked about Töbi more often now. Your thoughts were with him, even though he was far away in Tibet. You often said that you would have wished for a man like him in your life. There would be one problem: he would have to give up his vacations in high mountains. Even if you recovered, you would be unable to go with him.

"Dear Belli," I replied, "you must not do that. Either you will go with him or you will let him go by himself."

"All right, Mom, then I'll just visit you during that time!" you said.

You began to say goodbye more deliberately. Jan called you from Canada and asked you to hold out, at least until he came back. You had also promised Töbi that you would wait to die. That was the only thing that made you hold on. However, neither of them would come before the beginning of December. Would you make it until then? If you succeeded, why not stay alive until Christmas? But it would be sad to die in January, right after Christmas. In your hopes you were already well into the next year!

Since October 8, 1982, you had been writing in your diary for hours at a time and sometimes during the nights. You kept asking whether it bothered me. No, I was glad, because I knew the seriousness of your thoughts. You also told me that this diary was for us. On November 12 you talked about your great desire to write a letter to Töbi. Why shouldn't you write, I asked. "Well, mom, I love him, and if I don't die, I would like to marry him."

"Why not?" I said. "Before he left, he told me that he also liked you very much."

"But he has to wait until I'm twenty-five. First I have to graduate from college." The next night you began to write a letter to him.

In the middle of the night you asked me: "Mom, if God lets a miracle happen, and if I recover and reach age 25, would I then *have* to marry Töbi even if I had changed my mind?"

"Dear Belli, don't worry about that now. I know that Töbi has a big heart, and he would understand."

The next morning you wanted to talk to Matthias. You knew that your death would be very hard for him. For fourteen years of his life he had followed in your footsteps. You were only eighteen months apart. You always showed him the way. First he followed you to kindergarten, then to elementary school, and finally to high school. You also inspired him to play tennis and to jog. How would his life continue without you? Would he find his way on his own? You told me later that he talked to you about death and life after death.

I always left you alone at these personal farewells, even if I wanted to be with you. Matthias and you read Astrid Lindgren's *The Brothers Lionheart*. This enchanting story enabled you to share your thoughts. I was happy that I had read this book with you at a time when no one thought about illness and death. My reading to you and your reading on your own was bearing fruit. In these days

115

I started to read Michael Ende's *The Never-Ending Story* to you and to the boys whenever they were with you. The magic of the story blended with your own magic.

In the evening you talked to Dr. P. on the phone. This was a very deep conversation. She was not well either, and she had to expect the worst. Both of you made a date to meet in heaven.

At night you wanted to know how my parents died and how you would find them. I told you that my parents and Grandpa would be waiting for you at heaven's gate. We did not cry during these talks; we were very calm.

We sensed that these were your last days, and you wanted to see a few of your friends. You wanted to talk to Doris, Maren, Johannes, and Dorothea. Saturday Doris arrived from Oberursel. Later she wrote to you.

November 17, 1982

Dear Belli,

It was very, very good that we could meet Saturday. Unfortunately, Sunday did not work out.

I often think back to our last conversation. You asked me whether it bothered me. On the contrary, I'm happy about what you said, and I was really impressed by your faith. For the first time I saw how well, how very well, faith can carry a person. That's very good. And it is wonderful that you are content. Only very few people are happy like that, especially in a situation like yours.

Dear Belli, I hope you survive the pneumonia and that you will recover fully. With God nothing is impossible. Most

of all I hope you will be really happy and that you retain
your trust in God forever.

My warmest greetings,

Doris

P.S. Please give my heartfelt greetings to your family. My
mother sends her dearest wishes as well.

A Bible verse and a short saying come to my mind: "Let
us praise the God and Father of our Lord Jesus Christ, who
in Christ has blessed us with every spiritual blessing in
heaven" (Ephesians 1:3).

> *I asked God for all things,*
> *So that I could enjoy life.*
> *He gave me life instead*
> *So that I could enjoy all things.*

117

Johannes also came to visit you. I don't know much about these talks, except that they were very important to you. Maren couldn't make it on Sunday for health reasons. However, Hans-Jürgen came and brought you a bouquet of roses.

Dad stayed with you during the night from Sunday to Monday. You really needed to talk with him. A few days earlier you talked to me about how the family would carry on after your death. I told you that I worried how the boys would get along with Dad. Burdening you with this concern is the only thing I regret to this day. That really wasn't necessary.

When I came in Monday morning, neither one of you had slept very much. A lung X-ray was scheduled for that day to see whether the most recent treatments had accomplished anything. You wanted to make use of the time until then. First you had me write down who would get what of your things. Then you dictated a long entry for your diary. Good Lord, what I got to hear! Your words and your voice were so determined that I did not dare question you. I just wrote.

At eleven o'clock everything was prepared for the X-ray. For several days you had been sustained only by oxygen. Your bed was rolled to the radiology department to avoid any additional pain for you. During that time you had to be disconnected from the oxygen supply. It was estimated that you could get along without oxygen for fifteen minutes. Everything was prepared. The doors in the hallway were open; the elevator was ordered for an emergency trip; the radiology department awaited you. After fifteen minutes we were back in your room at the oxygen supply. Now we had to wait for the results. During that time you dictated several farewell letters to me.

A few days earlier you had a long conversation with Dr. Kern. I was with you. You asked him about your remaining options.

He said that it would depend. "If the analysis shows that the last Platinex therapy was successful, then you would receive further treatment."

"Okay, but if the last treatment did not produce any improvement, and the tumor is continuing to grow, then we don't have a chance?"

"That's right."

In the evening you saw everything much clearer. You seemed even set free and at times euphoric. You knew that your destiny was dependent on the results of the X-rays.

Soon the doctors and I knew about the outbreak of the metastases in your lungs. You did not ask about the results. There were still so many things to talk about and to arrange according to your wishes.

I went into the hallway for a few minutes, supposedly to get something from the kitchen. I talked to Dr. Petri, Dr. Kern, and the senior physician. "Should we inform Dr. Töbellius?" they asked. Had Isabell asked about the results already? She hadn't. For the first question, I had no answer. I asked the doctors: "Did Dr. Töbellius give you any instructions?"

"Yes."

"Has he requested to be informed if Isabell dies before he returns?"

"No, he hasn't told us anything about that."

"Then do not disturb him on his vacation. He needs his energies for other patients." I went back to your room.

You continued to organize your papers. At about two o'clock in the afternoon Dr. Kern came to see you. You asked him: "Do you have the results of the chest X-rays?"

"Yes."

"What are they?"

"Not good. The metastases have spread."

"Then I am resistant to the Platinex therapy too?"

"Yes."

"Then I don't want to be treated anymore. If God really wants to perform a miracle on me, he won't need chemotherapy. I put my life in God's hands. I'd like to talk to my parents."

Meanwhile I had called Dad. He was already on his way. You talked the details over with Dr. Kern. You wanted to die in dignity, without suffocating. And, if possible, you wanted to die without pain, so that your family wouldn't have to suffer so much. You were promised the alleviation of pain and that you would fall asleep quietly. How long it would take nobody could tell. The tumor would probably win out quickly once you stopped fighting.

Dad arrived. Dr. Kern informed him about the facts, and you asked Dr. Kern if we could be alone. You were firm in your decision: you did not want any new treatments. You had the final word. There was no leeway for contemplating, reconsidering, or even discussing. It was your life, and now only God should decide.

You asked us to stand together and be strong, not to fall apart as a family, to love our sons as we loved you, and to take care of Grandma. Meanwhile, we had also called Matthias, Christian, and Grandma. Christian came directly from work. In the hallway I told him everything. The doctors and nurses stood in front of your door. Nobody dared to ask anything.

This all happened too fast for Christian. He was not able to accept fate in that way. He asked the doctors and nurses to encourage you to begin a new treatment. That broke my heart. I became stubborn and said: "I will not let anyone go in Isabell's room who does not respect her decision!"

Christian pulled himself together. When you talked to him, he was calm. You asked him to accept your destiny and, facing him directly, you said: "I know that you have a difficult time ahead of you. You have your exam next week. I can't make it until then, even though I wish I could. Take the exam anyway, and try to pass. I'll help you. I'll sit on your shoulder and whisper in your ear. We won't be caught cheating!"

To Matthias you said: "Matthias, if you can, tell the people in school how I died. Perhaps they will have a funeral service for me. It would make me so proud if you could talk about my last hours."

You asked what time it was. 6:30 in the evening. You pulled out the letter to Töbi and added a few lines. You sealed it and asked us to give it to him together with a picture of a rose that you made. Then you said, "Dad and Mom, please get the doctors. They can start now."

They all were waiting outside your room. Dr. Petri and Dr. Kern had prepared everything for sedation. So, that was the purpose of the little box on wheels that we had seen in Cologne every now and then.

Your first question was: "Dr. Petri, will I die a natural death?"

"Yes, these sedatives will only put you into a deep sleep."

"Will I wake up once more?"

"No, not if you don't want to. You will sleep until death occurs."

"Will I have any pain?" you asked.

"As far as doctors know, there will be no pain."

You knew that you would die of suffocation, and you did not want to consciously suffer through this painful end.

"Please, Dr. Petri, go ahead." Dr. Petri adjusted the drip, held your left hand with his left, and with his right hand he felt your pulse. You were calm during this

121

whole time—almost happy—as if you were freed from a heavy burden. For the next forty-five minutes—until the very last—you talked very clearly to us.

"I wanted so much to see Dr. Töbellius one more time. He always had such a funny laugh. I was so presumptuous to have planned his whole life for him. I called him Töbi. Was it proper for me to do that? But after all, he was not just any Töbi, he was *my* Töbi!"

"Dr. Petri," you asked. "Why are so many people afraid of dying?"

Before he could answer, you replied. "Not everyone has such a wonderful family, such nice doctors, and such a good education as I have had!"

"Matthias, tear down the walls you encounter in life. And if you can't tear down the walls right away, make a hole and then try to make that bigger.

"Christian, take care of yourself. Whenever you have your first date, I will sit on your shoulder and whisper in your ear what you are supposed to say and do.

"Dad, be proud of your sons.

"Mom, you were my best friend.

"The four of you will now have a very good life. I will make sure of that. If there are problems, then I will have a little talk with God!"

Dr. Petri asked you: "Should I stop the procedure?"

"No, I am not changing my mind! I will now enter heaven happily. I am getting light and translucent, but I can see you.

"Dad, we have a date for 10:00 P.M., don't forget it." (Dad had promised he would always look at a certain star at ten o'clock to meet you there in thought.)

"Mom, when are we going to have our conversation each day?"

"At seven in the morning," I replied.

"Let's make it 6:00, when you're jogging. And with you, Christian?"

"At 7:00 P.M., when I come home."

"And Matthias, how about you?"

"At 6:30 when I get up."

"Dr. Kern?"

"That's easy, at twenty to eight, of course!"

"And Sister Ulrike?"

"At 6:30, when I arrive at the hospital."

"Tell Maren that dying is not hard. She should go to the hospital in Bonn. She is also going to die soon. I'm sorry that I couldn't see her again, but I didn't have the energy.

"Tell Dorothea that she should not feel bad about not visiting me last Saturday. I enjoyed Johannes' visit very much.

"Tell Siegfried and Ulli that my godchild made me very happy. They should have more children and they should become a healthy, happy family.

"I would have so much wished to see Jan and Töbi. I do like Jan more than I thought.

"I am tired and happy. I would rather have stayed with you. I will meet Grandpa. Mom, will your parents recognize me? They have never seen me. I will always be with you even if you don't see me anymore—especially when you are celebrating and when you are happy."

123

Your enunciation became unclear. I asked you to pray the Lord's Prayer with us. These sentences, spoken so often, were the last to come from your lips.

Your family gathered around you. The doctors and nurses left us alone with you. There was a holy silence. We were comforted by the thought that you had no pain anymore. Your breathing continued faintly with the oxygen.

The senior physician advised me to go home with the boys. Your unconsciousness could last for several days. I followed her advice. Paul and Hatty arrived to pick up Matthias, Christian, and Grandma, and they tried to comfort the boys at home. Siegfried arrived the same night from Mannheim.

Dad and I were alone with you. We hardly talked, but rarely had we been so close to each other. After a few hours Dad sent me home as well to get some sleep. He kept watch at your side with Sister Ulrike. You and Dad—I am sure—had a lot to tell each other in thought.

During these hours you were also closely connected to other people. Ines wrote a letter to you, not knowing about your condition.

NOVEMBER 16, 1982

My dear Isabell, you dear girl,

I think about you very, very often. I just want to tell you this. If only I could help you, I would give you every bit of energy I still have left. But I know that you have strength, inner strength and courage, and that you are bearing your illness in an exemplary manner. The love of your family and your friends will help you, but most important is what is within you. I know that you can cope with your destiny and that you will accept it.

I will pray for you.

Very gently I surround you with my thoughts.

Ines

öbi thought of you as well and wrote a postcard from Tibet dated November 15, the day you consciously bade farewell to us. The card arrived one day before your funeral. The card showed a boy next to an Indian elephant. I can recall the message only from memory, because we tucked the card underneath the flowers on your grave. I clearly remember the last part of a sentence: "Well, then I'll just become an elephant guide." Dr. Töbellius also mentioned that he hoped you wouldn't do anything silly.

The next morning Matthias and I came, and together we watched over your deep sleep. Dad could go home to rest for a few hours.

In the evening we were all together again. The sun was setting. We saw the Seven Hills and the lights from the Rhine. I took your diary and I started to read it aloud.

Belli's Diary

OCTOBER 8, 1982

I'm quite sad. I don't know why. Probably because I am in this stupid hospital in Cologne all by myself and because my ear aches. I am slowly getting fed up with this place. I have been here now for almost three weeks. Jacob hasn't called. He did call at home but not here. I would have liked it very much if he had called. Secretly I had hoped that he would stop by, but no such luck.

I have truly great parents. They were out with friends this evening. I called there, and Dad offered to come over right away. I am glad he's coming, and that he understood my need without my having to ask. That's so nice.

When I think about my right ear, it starts to hurt. So I mustn't think about it.

I believe that I could become good friends with Ingund. Whenever she is here, we have fun. My stupid right arm is hurting me. I hope it will get well sometime. Otherwise, I won't be able to play tennis anymore.

OCTOBER 16, 1982

Claudia is dead. Please, dear God, accept her in grace and reward her for her strength and her courage. I heard about it from Michael on Monday. I couldn't believe it at first. To me Claudia has always been a model patient, who would fight and defeat this illness. In June I hoped to accomplish what she did. Who would have ever guessed that this young woman, radiating with courage, would die so soon. Claudia gave me much courage when

I ran out of it and when I was hanging on by a thin thread. For me she was a role model because of her patience and determination. Now I have learned that she was not that way at the beginning and that she developed these qualities only toward the end when it was too late. But Claudia has certainly not died in vain. I at least hope I have learned from her mistakes, and I will try to become more patient and to follow the doctor's advice more closely. I do have the somewhat strange advantage of having pain whenever the tumor is growing. At least she died without agony within four days. She never had pain, and she tended to prolong the breaks between treatment and to discontinue the therapies so often. I hope that I will learn from her mistakes.

I always notice when the tumor is coming back because of the pain. That is a good warning signal, though it wears me down badly. For instance, yesterday my knee was hurting. I really should be grateful for the pain signal, but it is hard to be grateful for something so agonizing.

For the past few days I have felt more pain, and that depresses me. I had hoped that this treatment would have prolonged the time without pain. At first I was supposed to be treated in Cologne, but now I will be treated in Bonn.

I'm so happy about that. I wouldn't have wanted to go back to Cologne now.

Dr. Töbellius visited us at home today to talk everything over. All will work out well.

At 11:00 p.m. today Jan called me from Canada. He talked to me for almost fifteen minutes. I was very happy.

OCTOBER 18, 1982

Today was not so good until now. I have severe pain in my knee, and I had to take a heavy dose of painkiller, and that's why I am not all here. In my head I often see scary incidents: a girl drops down a ravine for fun, and at the bottom she is caught by a boy. Or a wall comes rolling toward me, and at the last moment it takes a turn. I experience all this very vividly, and that is why I feel threatened.

Earlier I felt discouraged, and I still do a little. I was frightened about the treatments. At such times I think I'm ugly, and I become pessimistic about everything.

Yesterday evening I thought of myself as pretty, and I was very calm, but later my calmness disappeared and I wanted to run away.

These stupid painkillers! I'm quite dizzy. Writing is hard for me. The pain is less though, and it's only in my knee.

I hope that something will be discovered soon to treat my knee effectively. This constant pain is really aggravating.

In the evening: The first day here in the Bonn hospital was not so good. I remembered the atmosphere differently. Almost all the nurses are new, and Dr. Kern did not come at all today.

I believe that I will have to keep myself busy while I'm here. I'm thinking a lot about nice Christmas presents for people. Maybe I could embroider something for Mom.

OCTOBER 19, 1982

Last night I did not sleep very well. I needed only one Fortral, but I woke up almost every hour. My knee is a terrible problem. If it doesn't get better soon, I may go to pieces. I feel half paralyzed. I also get upset when the nurses help only with silly little things, and not at all with the hard ones!

I do hope that my knee will get better at the beginning of the treatment. The infusion and the crutches scare me.

My dear Mom, I hope she will be back soon!

Today has changed much for the better. Mom dressed me and had breakfast with me. Then I went with Brigitte for the ultrasound, and after that Mrs. Martin came for an enjoyable and nice visit. Inge and Frau Keller came together. I unexpectedly had to go downstairs for X-rays. They were very careful and everything was done while I was in bed. That was incredibly considerate.

Finally I found a present for Matthias. Hatty gave me the idea. I will get him something from Nike. I still have to think of everything else.

O CTOBER   20,   1982

My parents and Dr. Töbellius think that I will die soon, because I cannot stand this difficult treatment anymore and because my knee is so bad. But I don't want to die. I don't feel like it at all. I know that I have become quite weak, but I don't want to die. Now the length of the treatment depends on me, but I don't want to give up yet. I just can't imagine how it would be not to live anymore. No, I simply must not die. My parents are so worried and scared. This morning, during my bath, Mom talked as if I wouldn't make it, and since then I've been shaking. I don't know why.

Not because I am afraid. The rear tip of my left lung hurts quite badly again. I don't want to die. I think it is just too dreadful to know every day that death is around the corner.

I just have to really want it. And I will, this afternoon, when the catheter will be inserted. The new treatment begins Friday.

There are three possibilities left for me: either the radiation treatment will make the pain go away; or the chemotherapy will finally be effective; or I will not be treated anymore, and then I will probably die.

I just talked about that to Frau Bell. I told her that I worry about my parents and my brothers, because they see less life in me every day.

At times, like just now, I'm flooded by waves of confidence, and then I'm certain that I can make it. Frau Bell talked to me about God, that he has so much power, and that we should trust in him. Perhaps Frau Bell is right. If I die, I would then be happy, and my family would be better able to accept it.

My goal was to make it to the end of December. I believe that now I will really have to show how much I want to live. There are still so many things I have planned. I just can't imagine that they won't happen anymore. At first in this illness death seems to come so slowly, but then it does occur very fast. Claudia also declined suddenly. Only two months ago I had the prospect of complete recovery—and now the situation looks quite different.

Mrs. Martin just called, and I cried on the phone. She wants to come by immediately. That's very nice. I hope we can communicate fairly well. It's so hard to talk about difficult topics without knowing the right words.

OCTOBER 21, 1982

They said that I would not have to suffer long if the chemotherapy was not successful. I'm afraid. I don't want to die. I can't imagine death, even though it is only one step away.

My pain is very bad. Even if I didn't want to fight anymore, the pain won't go away until death delivers me, the death I don't want. What choice do I have but to fight? Things can only get better. I can't imagine how it will be to know that I'm dying and to say goodbye to all my loved ones. I just don't want to die yet. Please, dear God, give me strength to make it. The next ten days will be unbelievably hard, but I just have to make it. I have to!

My right leg hurts so badly, and no one can do anything about it. I have terrible pains in my leg. My knee is so swollen, it will probably have to be drained once more. Today, when I talked to Dr. Kern, I learned that the treatment will only drain my knee. Now I am quite drowsy because of a Fortral shot earlier.

OCTOBER 22, 1982

Yesterday afternoon was very uncomfortable. Because of a painkiller my mind was gone the entire afternoon. I couldn't move, talk, or open my eyes decently anymore. Fortunately I managed to have this medicine discontinued, so I did feel better in the evening.

Emotionally I am swinging from highs to lows. Right now I am in quite a good mood because my knee doesn't hurt so badly, and last night was all right. The radiation treatments seem to work quite well. I think that I can get through these ten days!

I'm doing all right again. I also received wonderful news from Jan. He always wears a beret now in Canada, because he wants to look like me. He told Theresa that he likes me very much, although I had a different impression last summer. He would like to see me again. Perhaps they both will come back the beginning of December.

OCTOBER 23, 1982

The pains are worse again, especially in my tail bone. I'm so afraid I'm dying, because there isn't really any improvement. I become more and more aware of what it means to be seriously ill. The thought that I might never see the people I love anymore makes me very sad. If I die, it will certainly happen before Christmas. Yesterday I was so confident, but now I can't imagine a

131

bearable future anymore. Even death would be painful. But I don't want to die yet. There are still so many things I would like to do. I would like to see Jan and Theresa, and I would like to celebrate Christmas in the Black Forest. I just don't want to die yet.

I don't think I have the strength to fight against the pain much longer if this treatment doesn't bring any improvement. Then I might just have to continue living like a vegetable, stuffed with painkillers.

It would be easier to die if the moments before death could be pleasant and without pain, so that I could fully enjoy that time with my loved ones. All I know now is that death will increase my pain—and I hope for one more improvement with each agonizing treatment, at least until I die.

The wave of pain has passed, and now I feel all right again. Earlier I had a great conversation with Mom. Dad, on the other hand, seems very tense.

Marie will be here soon. I feel like I'm on a roller coaster. At the moment I am feeling all right again. I ate, and I didn't get sick.

I thank you, dear God, that you improved my emotions. This morning I was so afraid about death. Marie was very happy with the scarf. I think she was very moved as well; we both were a bit inhibited.

I also would like to be bathed again. Right now I'm sure I can make it. Fear of death is something really dreadful. I had fear, such great fear.

What makes me very happy is the concern of Frau Bell and Frau Niefindt. Both have offered to see me at any time. I am very curious to see if my emotions will continue to be on a roller coaster ride, and whether the second day of treatment will bring any significant help. Pain keeps coming in waves.

It is 9:00 p.m., and I feel quite well again. Just this morning I thought that I would never again feel all right. That tells me once more that I should never give up hope. And Töbi will be here tomorrow. I look forward to seeing him. Mom went to the tennis banquet tonight. I hope that she and Marie are having fun!

OCTOBER 24, 1982

Today began wonderfully. Marlene bathed me, and I had no pain. I didn't sleep all that well last night, but I'm sure that I'm going to make it.

Today the whole day was beautiful. Marie, Christian, and Mom visited for a long time, and before that Rolli came by (he is now staying in Cairo). Mrs. Martin and Töbi may come to see me too. Matthias certainly will.

My pain is under control, and I think my leg is getting better. I am prepared for a very long stay this time at the Bonn hospital. I believe that will give us more and better chances to get things under control quickly. During these treatments I'm able to eat and drink without getting sick, and that is incredibly pleasant. I am also very responsive and alert. I'm quite curious about what will happen to me. At least I can learn something in these days. My memory has been affected by all the treatments.

133

OCTOBER 25, 1982

Today I don't feel like writing very much, I just want to report the following: Today went by fast. I had visits from Frau Bell, Grandma, and Mom. Dad stayed overnight. He helped me analyze a dream, and that was really interesting.

OCTOBER 27, 1982

Yesterday was a stupid day. There were a lot of visitors—it was just too much. Inge came unannounced and brought me a few books about life after death. Dad found that quite inappropriate, and I certainly won't read them.

Yesterday Jacob called. That really surprised me, because I did not expect it at all. He said that he will stop by.

In the evening Christian visited me. He was so dear and sweet. He is really okay, after all.

Sister Ulrike is also incredibly nice. She gave me two photos of the doctors at the Bonn hospital and one of Töbi. I believe she is the nicest nurse I ever had. This morning she suggested that I give Dr. Kern a wake-up call, which I did. It was a lot of fun.

OCTOBER 31, 1982

Dad writes me sweet little stories. Here is one of them: Once upon a time there was a dwarf. He was upset because his feet were very very big. He prayed: "Dear God, give me smaller feet." And a miracle happened. At Christmas Santa Claus brought him small slippers, and when the dwarf put them on, his big feet fit nicely into the little slippers. His other wish, however, to become a tall human being, was not granted. He is still praying.

And another one: A little girl saw a star twinkling in the sky. "Are there any humans on that star?" she asked.

Her father thought about it. "Yes. They are very small, have crooked legs, are green, and have egg-shaped heads with antennas."

"Oh, then they look just like my brother when he gets angry!!" said the little girl, quite pleased.

NOVEMBER 4, 1982

I believe I have won a small victory again. I feel much stronger, I am hungry again, and I can walk.

I like Dr. Töbellius very much. I think he likes me too. Today he said goodbye for the third time. He is leaving for Tibet to go mountain climbing. He told Mom that never before has he felt so close to a young patient. Mom and I talked for a long time yesterday evening, and she thought that at the age of twenty-five, I would be a quite adequate partner for him. I would like to marry him. That thought makes me happy. We both understand one another so well.

Today Dr. Burbi came to say goodbye to me. I also get along very well with him and Dr. Kern.

My so-called "embolism of the lung" was only a reaction to the high dosage of Dipidolor.

I'm quite anxious about what will happen on Sunday with Jacob. I am also eager for my Christmas blankets to arrive.

NOVEMBER 5, 1982

I just took a bath and enjoyed it very much. Earlier I called Bertin, and I asked him if I could have a recording. He must have changed quite a bit. His voice was very low, and he was being quite cool.

This morning Pastor Muller came by again. I asked him why he came unannounced. His visit was quite annoying.

Today is Töbi's first day of vacation. I feel bad that I won't see him for such a long time.

Siegfried, Ulli, and Sascha will arrive tomorrow. They probably partied last night, and so are too tired to visit today.

Tomorrow Herr Kirchstein—pardon me, Friedrich—will visit me again. He scolded me for not calling him by his first name. Today Matthias will meet Friedemann. Dad and Matthias went to Berlin yesterday.

NOVEMBER 6, 1982

Today was a nice day. Sascha, Siegfried, and Ulli were here—and Sascha is so sweet.

I also ate a scoop of ice cream today, my first in a long time. Now I usually have an amazing appetite.
Tomorrow will also be great. Johannes, Dad, Matthias, and Jacob will come to visit. I wonder how it will go.
Unfortunately I can't write much because my arm hurts. Everyone is very pleased with my progress. Next week I will start to get out of bed again, in order to pick myself up and recover. In two weeks I would like to buy many beautiful things.

NOVEMBER 7, 1982

Matthias and Dad, together with Mom and Christian, were here a little while ago. They had funny things to say about their trip to Berlin. Fidi will come on Wednesday. I look forward very much to that because I really like her. I wonder how it will be when Jacob comes. He called again this afternoon, when I was puttering around. He said that he had a little cough; but since my leuko count is up to 1900 again, that shouldn't be serious.

When Töbi comes back I definitely want to ask him for a photo of himself. I do have pictures from Ulrike, but in them you can hardly recognize Töbi. I would rather have pictures from him.

Jacob was here from 4:30 to 6:00. That was nice. We had a very stimulating conversation, mostly about love and friendship. I think that he has many female friends and that he has had experience in bed.

According to Jacob, I have a good figure and a pretty face. I imagine that flirting with him would be quite nice. At least I think it's very kind of him to go through the trouble of visiting me all the way from Aachen.

He also had the impression that I would enjoy flirting and that I would do that quite well. At least he treats me like a woman and not like a girl. Töbi treats me more like a girl, but he's also much older. It is very interesting indeed to get to know men, and it is fun to flirt with them.

Jacob will be back in Cologne next Monday. Then we would like to get in touch again. Today he stroked my cheek when he said goodbye. I wonder how daring he will be in the future.

NOVEMBER 9, 1982

Yesterday was Matthias' birthday. I was allowed to leave the hospital for the afternoon. It felt wonderful to be home again. I believe that Matthias was really happy about that—Christian and my parents too.

It was a really beautiful and cozy afternoon at home. But last night I realized how much energy this visit cost me. I couldn't sleep, because my muscles ached so badly. I was quite desperate, and I had to take a Fortral.

Sometimes—like right now—I get very scared about whether I will make it. The pain is back again, but I can't tell what kind of pain it is, just a muscle ache or maybe something more serious. Now I feel really weak. Walking exhausts me. I'm out of breath immediately. Will this ever change? Last night Mom brought me here to my bed and hugged me. At that moment I felt very small again and in need of protection. It is good to know that I can be like that.

I feel awful right now. I am afraid that I won't make it. Everything hurts, and I don't feel well. Good that Mom will be here soon.

NOVEMBER 10, 1982

I'm at a low spot again. I caught a bacterial cold. This morning I was so scared because I thought that my fever was caused by the tumor—and that would have meant it's growing, in spite of the treatments. However, that is not the case. They found an infection. This also is very dangerous for me, because I could die of it. But I absolutely want to make it, because I promised Dr. Töbellius I'd behave.

This morning I mentally wrote some farewell letters. I thought about how I could finish my Christmas shopping, because I want to give a little happiness to others. I was just about ready to give up, because I was so scared.

I am in no way out of danger yet. Because my leuko count is so low, I could die quickly. This morning my temperature was 104.2 degrees Fahrenheit. Now I am back to 100.9 thanks to Novalgin and compresses around my calves. Dr. Kern has also removed my catheter and inserted a new one in my left arm. He wanted to make sure that the end of the catheter was not infectious.

This morning Dad was just as scared as I was. His eyes were very watery. He too had probably thought about my dying soon.

I want to forget this incident as soon as possible. I will certainly not be able to get out of here now, but I can deal with that. This morning I thought about writing letters to a few people. Funny, how changeable my confidence is. Just three hours ago I was ready to give up, and now I'm very relaxed about everything. I think I just wet my bed. The pee just ran out.

It would make me very happy if Marlene could give me a bath this afternoon and if she would change my sheets. I'm sure that I'll be able to wash myself soon because the catheter and the container from above have been removed.

Mom just came with ice cream and french fries.

This evening I had a very honest conversation with Dr. Kern. Until now I always had illusions. I thought that the Platinex therapy was *the* way of healing and that I would recover after only a few treatments. Today I learned that the therapy is only partially effective and that the condition of my lungs hasn't improved at all. Also my arm hurts badly.

The Platinex therapy is therefore not the miracle treatment, and the more often it is applied, the more resistant I become. That means that my chances will gradually diminish and that I will probably die soon. When Dr. Kern destroyed my illusions, I was really shaken. But still this was a good thing. In a way I'm even pleased and happy now. Everything is settled, and I have a clear perspective. That doesn't at all mean that I have given up. On the contrary, I don't believe that the infection will set me back very much. The pain will get worse though, and the next treatment won't produce a miracle either.

Dr. Petri and Dr. Kern saw me again this evening, and both of them told me that I don't need to be worried about suffering pain. That makes me quite happy.

If I really wanted to live on, I could prolong my life for about a month even without treatment—only with radiation, painkillers, and Cortisone.

I absolutely want to live as long as possible to make destiny easier to bear for my loved ones.

I feel more pleasantly tired and comfortable than I have for a long time. I simply don't think about dying. I feel so strong.

Dad and Mom just left for home, but Mom will be back shortly.

For a little while, Dad and I talked fondly and affectionately. For the first time in a while we kissed each other on the mouth. In the past—when I was small—that seemed natural, but it has a different meaning for me now, something for people in love.

I am too tired, my eyes don't see clearly, and my hand doesn't want to move anymore. I look forward to tomorrow. I mustn't forget to give Dr. Kern a wake-up call!

NOVEMBER 11, 1982

One year ago today I was admitted to the hospital in Bonn. It was very early in the morning, at 2:33 a.m. Being full of painkilling drugs is a strange feeling. I'm really quite tired, but still I can't sleep. My situation really worries me. Right now I can't even think about it logically. I would like to get rid of something so much, but I don't even know what it is.

I have a very bad conscience, because I don't let Mom sleep.

My dear parents, I thank you a thousand times that you take care of me so devotedly. I love you forever and I will always be with you.

Right now I am in a very melancholy mood. I can't figure out whether or not this mood is pleasant. I am basically incredibly tired, and my eyes fall shut, but when I lie down, I can't sleep. I just can't imagine not being around much longer. I really wanted to enjoy my life: flirt with boys and men, discover love, and then get married. I would have so much wanted to marry Töbi, because with him I feel safe, and we understand each other so well, even without words.

I have still one wish in this life: I would like to see Töbi one more time, and I want him to hold me and comfort me. I would so much like to continue living, but I don't believe that a miracle will save me.

I am too tired. I will stop now and ask God to give me sweet sleep and a pleasant dream. Please, dear God, grant me that favor.

I'm going back and forth between being very happy and very sad. I became quite confused after talking to Dr. Kern, although everything seemed so clear at the time. Most of the time when he talks to me, I end up crying.

Just now six children came in to sing St. Martin songs. It made me incredibly happy but at the same time

I was very sad. I had to cry a lot because the songs awakened so many memories. Claudia and Brigitte comforted me so nicely.

The best time to die would really be at the beginning of January. By then I would have celebrated Christmas, seen Töbi and Jan, and prepared for everything emotionally. If my dying is drawn out longer than three months, it would be so hard for everyone.

NOVEMBER 12, 1982

It's very early in the morning and I am keeping Dad from sleeping again. I absolutely believe in a miracle. Why shouldn't I make it? Yesterday evening Kiki and Brigitte stopped by, and Kiki was very moved. I like her more and more.

Why shouldn't I get over this damn cancer? I want to give everything I have, and I will show it! I love my parents so much, and I would so much like to give them my victory as a Christmas present.

I'm so afraid of getting pneumonia. Then I would die before Töbi and Jan return. Dad just got me some Fanta (at five in the morning). He is so loving. I don't want to lose him!

I do have pneumonia. There's a chance that I'll get over it, but it is quite unlikely that I will continue to live. Right now I have no more motivation to go through a Platinex therapy for the third time. I'm afraid to subject myself to such an ordeal. Earlier I announced to everyone that I had the will to live, but now I want to give up like a coward. In any case, I'll try to survive the pneumonia, and then everything will depend on the amount of time I have left. If I'm still alive in December—even without treatment—and have a few days with Töbi and Jan, I would not want to have anymore treatments, unless I have a chance of getting better. But I won't think about this anymore until I have recovered from the pneumonia. Whenever I talk to Marlene about the treatment of my dead body, she only giggles. Mom thinks that Marlene is very much afraid of death herself.

I can certainly talk about that with Töbi. I would also like to ask him whether donating my dead body would be helpful. I would so much like to reveal my feelings to him. But I don't know if he wants that. I would love to cuddle up with him and find comfort. Would he like that? Will I have enough strength to talk at all and to hug him?

Dear God, please grant me this one great wish: let me see Töbi while I am still fully conscious.

I simply refuse to stop believing in a miracle. Why shouldn't I make a super recovery from the pneumonia and still have enough energy to get through a third Platinex therapy? And why shouldn't it be successful? And if it brought some improvement I would gain new courage, and I would try out further Platinex treatments.

Astrid just visited me. I may now call her by her first name. We share the same birthday. I wanted so badly to become seventeen years old, and suddenly I was motivated by the wish to live longer. It would be so sad to die at Christmas—right after receiving so many gifts. Perhaps a strong will and a therapy to which I respond will achieve more than all the medication.

At least, the doctors just told me that I am doing much better. So the medication is working, and at the moment I feel quite well. Tomorrow Dr. Kern and Dr. Petri have a day off, but they want to visit me anyway.

I just talked to Matthias about death. That gave me a very beautiful and happy feeling. He told me to imagine heaven the way it is described in the book *The Brothers Lionheart*, and that death can be something beautiful.

I was very happy during this time, and then Dr. Burbi visited me as well. He was incredibly kind. He promised to support my decisions, also regarding therapy, if I want to give up.

Then I had physiotherapy, and I managed to cough up mucus. That made me very happy. I was, however, quite exhausted after that. My elated feeling has diminished a bit now; I must have overexerted myself when I was coughing. My right hand is shaking a lot, as can be seen in my handwriting. I can't put any weight on my left knee anymore, but I'm not supposed to worry about that. I can move my right arm in every direction again. I still do believe in a miracle. Thank you, dear God!

I received Björn's photos, and I don't think they're any good at all—but he does. I think I will write a reassuring letter to him.

Now I will rest.

I just talked to Mrs. P. on the phone. Now I talk to her informally, and we had a very deep conversation. She was given the wrong blood and is doing badly. She would like to die, and she believes in *a human life* as I do (as in *The Brothers Lionheart*). Mrs. P. said that she is still in contact with her son who died some time ago. I promised to call her often. She is suffering a lot now. During my normal life I was never as happy as I am now.

NOVEMBER 13, 1982

This morning I wasn't happy at all, even though I had slept quite well. I was so confused and unsure about my feelings. I was hungry as a horse and ate the upper halves of two rolls. Then I did feel better. I also started the letter to Töbi, and I really have a lot to say to him. Doris visited me at 11:00, and our deep conversation made me very happy. In that moment I was tremendously overjoyed and calm. I was also breathing much better. After I offered, she agreed to have her letters from our correspondence back. Now I feel quite energetic. The senior physician told me that I would not die of heart failure, although my heart rate is quite rapid.

It feels strange when I ask people which gifts would make them happy, because I'm thinking about my death. If I stay alive, it would really be embarrassing. But I have completely surrendered myself into God's hands.

One of Dad's stories of a little girl: It is just before Christmas. The little girl is curious about her presents.

"Dad, I will get a lot of presents, won't I?"

"Yes, my dear. You'll get a lot."

"Oh, that's great, I will get a lot. But Dad, how much is a lot?"

"Oh, this and that and then some."

"What, that much? I'll get so much—this and that and then some! And the boys will only get this. I really look forward to Christmas."

Jan has just called from Canada. That made me so happy. I promised him I'd stay alive until he returns. He sounded very sweet. I still like him very much.

I just said goodbye to Björn and thanked him for the photos. I'm curious how he will take the farewell. Johannes was just here too, and he stayed for an hour and a half. We ended our conversation only because Dad came in and wanted to know whether the visit was getting too much for me. He got "no" for an answer, and he seemed angry when he left the room. At the end, Johannes shook my hand with both of his, very sweetly, and I believe it wouldn't have taken much for him to hug and even kiss me. He told me that I am very important to him and that he never had such a conversation about death. I like Johannes very much. He would like to visit me once more. Of all the boys my age, I like him the best.

We talked about friendship, a respectful sexual relationship, and our ideas of eternal life. I told him that I once had a crush on him. He already experienced having a crush on a girl too. I would have never believed that.

I have the very strong feeling that I will get well again. But I am afraid of the treatments. Perhaps a miracle will happen, and I will get well through my willpower. Please, dear Lord, help me do this. I'm as stubborn as a mule!

11:30 p.m.: With Dad's help I have managed to cough up a lot of mucus. A great success!

NOVEMBER 15, 1982

I'm unable to write down my thoughts, because the radiation treatment of my right arm had to be discontinued over the weekend. Mom will fulfill my wish by writing down the thoughts about these last days, because I trust her unconditionally and because I gave my parents permission to read my diary after my death.

Saturday evening I again managed to get rid of a lot of mucus with Dad's help. Then we thought we would spend a quiet night. But that was not the case. We had a very long, honest, and difficult conversation. A few evenings earlier I promised Mom I'd talk to Dad about the touchy situation between him and the boys. I gave Mom that promise, because she felt misunderstood and treated unfairly by all three men of her family. That was on the evening before their trip to Berlin. In part I shared her opinion, and in any case I wanted to help her.

So I asked Dad what he would say if I told him that his sons were having problems with their father. He wanted to know in what way, and I gave him examples. One of them was that Dad could not stand any competition between him and his sons. He became quite angry and said that these were all empty phrases that I must have heard from Mom. I was quite hurt. I did not want to lecture him; I just wanted to open his eyes a little. I apologized for not being very good at telling him such things and also for using arguments that were not necessarily my own. I asked him not to be angry at me; I just did not want to pass on this task to the boys when I died; that would depress me a great deal. He said that he loved the boys very much and that I need not worry. I asked him to try hard for a close relationship with his sons after my death, because that would make me very happy.

I also told him that I would be able to see everything from heaven and that I would always be with him in thought. We promised always to think of each other and in that way be together every evening at 10:00 p.m. I also explained to him that he should experience the time of mourning as a very valuable time with his beloved wife. If two people lose the child of their love, the pain can only bring them closer to one another.

During this night we didn't sleep much anymore, and the next day we suffered the consequences.

I was being washed and I ate well, but then I had unbearable pain in my arm. This was shortly before 10:00, and Dr. Kern was not there yet. The doctor on duty came in and gave me a very strong dose of painkiller. My fears came true, and I suffered another setback. This time I fortunately had myself under control quite well, so I did not choke. But I was very scared. I hadn't yet prepared anything in the event of my death. Physically the situation was extremely uncomfortable for me. Sister Claudia proved her strength in a crisis and calmed me down by extensively rubbing Transpulmin on me for over an hour. Meanwhile Dr. Kern was master of the situation again and administered a tranquilizing solution. Dad rubbed my feet so that I slept for two and a half hours soon after that. Fortunately nobody telephoned. If they had, Dad would have eaten the person alive!

At 2:30 p.m. the changeover took place, and Mom came in. Dad went home to recover from the shock. While Mom was here, I dictated a kind of last will and testament to her. I wanted to give joy to a few good friends by leaving certain things to them. All that will be put down in more details in my diary. I still feel strong enough to live as long as I want to.

I had a quiet night with Mom. I slept for seven hours—but with interruptions.

his was the end of your diary.

You wrote a few farewell letters to the loved ones you did not get to see again during your last days. You did not expect Grandma to be there in your last hour, so you wrote to her.

November 15, 1982

Dear Grandma,

My dearly loved grandma. I may not get to see you any-more before I go to heaven. I will certainly meet Grandpa, and I won't have to tell him anything about us down here. In spirit I will continue to live with you. I don't want to die yet. I'm fighting very hard to stay with you. Perhaps God will still allow a miracle to happen. If time allows, I will write more to you.

I love you very much.

Your grandchild,

Belli

My precious Lou,

My will was not strong enough to tell you these words myself. You know how much I appreciated and loved your family. You gave me many happy hours. For that I thank you from the bottom of my heart. This letter is specially to you because I know that you, as a mother, will best know how to tell everyone individually what I have to say.

Please tell Caroline that she was as close to me as a sister. We communicated mainly through facial expressions and gestures, but it was always clear. I have rarely been hugged and kissed so nicely by any other friend. I will think about Caroline often, and I hope that she can feel my love every now and then.

I think Axel knows that I had a big crush on him for a long time. Maybe I was even in love with him. I still like him very much, and I hope that my affection meant something to him. It was beautiful and exciting to share loving glances with a boy. I often dreamed about Axel. Was I ever part of his dreams? At times I really wanted to know.

Dear Lou, and now about you. With you I feel a tie of deepest friendship. I have confided in you at all times. I hope that you will continue living happily for many years to come.

I don't know Manuell, Kati, and Albert enough to tell them much, but I liked them too. Hug them for me.

I feel very grateful and close to you.

Isabell

NOVEMBER 15, 1982

Dear Jan,

I respect you very much. Thank you for your fairness at all times.

Isabell

NOVEMBER 15, 1982

Dear Marie,

I love you like my own sister. It was beautiful to experience the feeling of having a sister. You have given me very much.
Till we meet again in heaven!

Belli

P.S. Greetings to your whole family, to the kitchen maid, and especially to your mother, who faithfully sent cards to me.

149

At the end of the diary was the sealed letter to Töbi. On the outside you wrote, "To my dear Töbi." Everyone looked eagerly at that letter. I took it in my hands and said: "Only Belli knows the content of this letter. It will remain a secret between Töbi and Belli." I closed the diary.

Dad, Matthias, Christian, and I kept watch at your bed for the rest of the night. During your last minutes we made a circle around you and held each other's hands. You bonded us forever. It was Prayer and Repentance Day, November 17, 1982, six o'clock in the morning when you were set free.

Siegfried, Ulli, and Grandma took the boys and comforted them.

We did our last duty. Just two days ago you gave me the instructions. You wanted to wear the white dress that you wore at Communion. And you wanted to have the pastel blue cotton scarf around your head. You wanted no wig, but also no bald head. And you asked for a big funeral. You said, "Everyone who wants to be at my funeral should be able to come." We didn't think we had energy, but you carried us, and we were encouraged by your strength.

We could even be supportive to others in the following days. You understood your death to be a new beginning, an exaltation, an honor! Friends who came to comfort us went home happy and enriched, because we told them about you—how you accepted your destiny without reservation, and how you bade farewell to life, being reconciled to everything. Such a farewell was possible because we were all honest with you, and also because there was harmony between the doctors, you, and us; we told you about all the results whenever possible by having conversations with you and the doctors together. That allowed you to share your thoughts, fears, and hopes with us. This was the essential prerequisite that enabled you to accept your death. For many people you set a wonderful example.

Apart from the fact that you were not with us anymore physically, we had no reason to be sad. That protective and wondrous comfort was incredibly strong during the first days. We were proud of having had such a daughter and sister. You fulfilled your destiny, you lived your life, even though it seemed to be so short.

Thanks to you we were able to spend this time intentionally and creatively, not simply as victims. This was a uniting and essential experience in our lives.

You accepted what was unavoidable in your life; everything else you always took into your own hands and tried to shape it positively. You are a shining example to many people who knew you; and you will become a shining example to many, many readers—after only sixteen and a half years of life!

The funeral—nine days later—was held after Christian's exam. He, and certainly you too, gave your best. He passed in spite of all the burdens. He came straight from his exam to church for the funeral service. You had asked for Matthias' confirmation pastor, but you wanted the funeral to be in our church, where you had been confirmed.

It was a grand farewell. On this day we clearly saw how many people loved you. We were your parents and brothers, and that filled us with great pride. From now on we wanted to try especially hard, so you could be proud of us too.

At the school memorial service Matthias gave his first speech. In your last hour you had asked him to tell his schoolmates about how you died. "I promised her," Matthias reported at the service in the school chapel, "and she told me that no one needs to be afraid of dying. She was absolutely sure that she would continue to live and that we would meet again. In the evening Isabell went to heaven, gently, relieved, and happy." You must have been very proud of him.

The expressions of sympathy were overwhelming—in school and from all our friends and acquaintances. For example, you would be interested in the obituary written by your tennis coach for the club paper:

> Isabell Zachert is no longer alive. She was only sixteen years old. For one year doctors, and especially she herself, fought against a most malicious illness. Between anxiety and hope, Isabell defended herself defiantly, even doggedly against the threatening end. She knew that it was coming.
>
> A break between treatments at Pentecost gave her the last opportunity to visit the tennis club, her "home" in sports. We love to remember her report in the club paper, in which she cheerfully described her impressions about the last tournament. Several times she was club champion in her division. She was a cheerful person, always cooperative and

willing to help. She once gave promise of becoming a good junior player, and in her last week she told me quietly and sadly, "Now I'm probably a loss for the tennis club."

Isabell, we really miss you—forever.

SIBYLLE PAGENKOPF

Dr. L. gave us a poem he had written about you:

You showed us death
  and life
    by walking ahead of us.
      You left your loved ones
        to follow a dark and forbidding path.
          Your eyes saw ahead
            and grew wise.
          You are an example
            to all who will die.
              You are not forgotten.
            Isabell,
              you live on.

153

After the funeral, following your instructions, we drove to Altglashütten in the Black Forest, to Gerda and Ernst.

It took us quite some time to realize how tense we were. If on this trip we had all gone directly to heaven, we wouldn't have minded. We all wanted so much to be with you. Being in such a condition is a particularly dangerous time for accidents to occur. Fortunately you took good care of us.

Life went on. According to your own wish, we spent your small "fortune" by going out to the Maternus Wine House with Grandma. As you promised, you were with us in spirit. That was the first time we were out in public again. It was our twenty-first wedding anniversary!

My dear Isabell, I will resist the temptation to tell you everything that happened since then. You know it anyway. But I have to mention a few important events. After all, it's possible that you have flirted too much in heaven so that you were distracted every now and then!

Maren died four months after you in the Bonn hospital, just as you predicted in your farewell hour. From now on we parents—Inge, Hans-Jürgen, and Dad and I—imagine you two girls together, jumping around without crutches or wheelchairs.

Your godmother Ines died two years after you. When she went to the hospital for the last time, she called me to Munich, so that I could be with her and her daughters.

A few days ago I met Michael, the student from the clinic in Cologne who had a tumor. Ten years after his treatment in Cologne he introduced me to his wife and his three-year-old son. I was so overjoyed that I hugged him spontaneously: "Michael, you conquered the tumor!"

Two weeks ago I talked to Dr. P. and told her about my plan to write this book. She said to me: "You have to do it, and you will!" She was just on her way to the hospital for another operation.

The love of our children and friends carried us through. Dad and I found ourselves and each other again. During the entire time we both had lived in a partnership with you. Now we had to understand that we could and had to relate to each other again—and also to Matthias and Christian. In this world we lost our daughter, but we kept our two wonderful sons. You wanted us to be a cheerful and happy family after your death. You managed to accomplish that: we have become happy. And because we are, we can successfully go on our individual ways.

My dear little Belli, I am sitting in Somme-Leuze on the balcony, and I'm dreaming. Our work will succeed! Yesterday Dad came to visit me in the Ardennes. It rained hard, but we sat cozily by the fireplace. I read to him everything I had put down on paper so far, drawn from the refreshing well of memories. Fortunately I did not get lost in the valley of tears.

He was very moved and grateful. I am filled with joy. With every day of writing I became more at peace. This emerging book is only the necessary supplement to your letters and your diary. It is your book, and it will be a little memorial to you. You fully deserve this. For me this is keeping an unspoken promise to you. Your life and your suffering were deeply meaningful. You have not died in vain. You are a model to everyone who knew you in life, and now you will become a model to many more. The problem of death is a question every person faces in life. The fear of taking a stand is great. You will help many people in doing that. For me personally, you are a model for the rest of my life.

It is Sunday noon. The bells are ringing in Somme-Leuze. These have been ten wonderful days with you. But before I return to everyday life, I have to talk something over with you: "What do you want me to do with

Töbi's letter?" Töbi gave me the letter before I left for the Ardennes. He said: "If you write a book about Isabell, you will also have Belli's letter." That was the decision of our friend Töbi. What do you think? Do you want readers to believe that your destiny was fulfilled? In the letter to Töbi you provide the answer yourself: "I give courage to so many people, and perhaps my radiant happiness will take away their fear of death."

NOVEMBER 13, 1982

My dear Dr. Töbellius,

I want to share my innermost feelings with you, and I want to do that honestly, because I know that now I won't be able to bother you with these feelings anymore.

I dare to write all this to you, because I think that you will at least understand and perhaps find some joy as well.

I promised you I'd stay out of trouble while you were gone. I'm very sorry that a complication occurred after all, but I promise you that I will use all of my willpower to hold out at least until you come back.

Maybe your presence will give me enough energy to hold out even longer, so that we will have some time for each other.

At least my feeling tells me that I can make it.

My most beautiful moments of the day were your visits, when I could see you every day.

During the night I often dreamed about how wonderful it would be if you felt the same affection for me that I feel for you.

It may sound arrogant for a young girl like me to suppose that a mature man would be interested in her. I am fully aware that I cannot yet be a partner for you. Intellectually I could never offer you satisfying conversations.

But in my dreams I always wished that you would become a close friend with our family after my recovery. And with the years I could become more interesting to you until I could be your match in important matters.

That was a beautiful dream of mine, and I know that it is farfetched. That is why I never dared to touch the bubble containing my dream, for fear that it would burst.

As I wrote in the beginning of this letter, I want to hold out by all means until you come back, but unfortunately I have no guarantee of that. That is why I am writing down my thoughts of you, and I hope that they will convey something of my love, my confidence, my deepest respect, and great admiration.

Often I long to cuddle up with you. I dream that you hold me and give me strength.

I have painted a picture for you, a rose with a tiny bud. The big, beautiful, vigorous rose is you, and I am the little bud looking for your protection. The leaf has no further meaning. It is only to fill out the space in the picture.

If I have to die, which is very likely but not altogether certain, there is only one thing I would have missed in my life on earth: to have loved and married a man. I don't know whether this thought pleases you, but I imagined a wonderful marriage with you.

Please forgive these bold remarks. It helps me greatly to share my most intimate feelings without having them weigh too heavily on you. Nobody will know about the content of this letter, not even my parents, although I have complete trust in them.

I just don't know how pleasant or unpleasant my feelings are for you, and that is why you are the only one who knows.

157

I am not afraid of death. You, Dr. Petri, and Dr. Kern took away all my fears about pain, and I've never been as happy as during these last days.

This is surprising to many, because other people are quite depressed and fearful about death; but I believe in a life hereafter and that it will correspond to the life of my dreams. There I may experience the love of a man, and I am also ready to wait for you and to listen to your feelings.

However, I really intend to be alive when you come back. Perhaps you will be embarrassed to see me then, after I have openly told you about all my feelings. You don't need to worry though. I don't want this letter to put you under any pressure.

I will not mention my letter, and I will leave it up to you whether or not to bring it up.

You are and will remain a free man. I simply wanted to share my feelings, hoping they would make you happy. You once told my mother that you liked me a lot. That is why I thought that my words would make you happy.

My will to live until you return is incredibly strong. I promised you I'd stay out of trouble. So I don't want you to blame yourself for not being here if I die.

I do believe in miracles, however. Why shouldn't the cancer be defeated when it sees my will to live? I am very reluctant to go through the suffering brought on by another treatment, because the chance of recovery is too small. God will either let me live without treatment, or he will let me die in spite of treatment.

I have the unconditional will to live, but I do not fear death. If these indeed are my last days, then they certainly were my happiest.

I often wondered why such a likable and unusual man like you does not have a wife. Perhaps life in the hospital is so fulfilling for you that you don't need a wife. This actually made me a little sad, because that would mean you wouldn't need me either.

Please don't think of me as presumptuous and conceited for revealing such a high opinion of myself. I just feel so strong, full of life and love that anything else would be dishonest.

If my wish comes true after all, and I see you once more, that would be wonderful.

Then there would be no misunderstandings, and I would feel sheltered in your presence. I would cuddle up with you very closely and be alone with you.

It would give me the greatest joy if you would hold my hand in the hour of my death. I pray to God that you will not misunderstand my letter and that you won't feel bothered and think of me as an immature child.

I believe that you are still young enough to be able to accept my feelings. Right now I feel tremendously strong, and I have no pain. I think of my illness and my crisis as a gift of God.

I give courage to so many people, and perhaps my radiant happiness will take away their fear of death.

NOVEMBER 15, 1982, 6:30 P.M.

I longed so much to see you one more time. We will meet again in heaven.

My deepest love.

Your Isabell,
Your little Isabell

We thank all the friends who shared our
burden, and all those who helped us accept it.

CHRISTEL AND HANS ZACHERT,
CHRISTIAN AND MATTHIAS